Research shows that training in specific techniques and theories contributes little to effective psychotherapy outcomes. What are well-intentioned clinicians who want to improve their skills to do? Read *The Field Guide to Better Results*. This book offers readers a practical roadmap to making their sessions more successful and enjoyable while helping them grow as therapists (and as people). I highly recommend this book.

—PAUL J. LESLIE, EdD, AUTHOR OF *THE ART OF CREATING A MAGICAL SESSION:
KEY ELEMENTS FOR TRANSFORMATIVE PSYCHOTHERAPY*

One of the biggest questions facing practicing clinicians today is how to improve and personalize psychological interventions based on the available research literature. This outstanding book will teach readers how to tackle this important task and how to develop their clinical skills further. It provides the necessary research basics as well as deliberate practice training examples to improve treatment options and make use of available monitoring tools. Comprehensive and fun to read, this volume helps to move the practice of psychological therapy forward.

—WOLFGANG LUTZ, PhD, DEPARTMENT OF PSYCHOLOGY,
UNIVERSITY OF TRIER, TRIER, GERMANY

This field guide offers a user-friendly path on how to engage in deliberate practice in order to achieve better treatment outcomes. The authors provide detailed exercises on how to become more effective psychotherapists. Kudos!

—DONALD MEICHENBAUM, PhD, RESEARCH DIRECTOR OF THE MELISSA INSTITUTE FOR VIOLENCE
PREVENTION AND TREATMENT, CORAL GABLES, FL, UNITED STATES

An eminently original, engaging, and practical book that draws together the latest research findings to help therapists of all orientations improve their work. "Deliberate practice" is a major new innovation in the training and development of psychotherapists, and this field guide—written by leading figures in the psychotherapy world—provides unique, step-by-step guidance to applying its method and insights.

—**MICK COOPER, DPhil,** PROFESSOR OF COUNSELLING PSYCHOLOGY, UNIVERSITY OF ROEHAMPTON, LONDON, ENGLAND

This book offers a wonderful combination of state-of-the-art scientific evidence on what makes therapists effective, in understandable language, and hands-on exercises for clinicians to improve their effectiveness. It is truly unique in that sense!

—**KIM de JONG, PhD,** SENIOR ASSISTANT PROFESSOR OF CLINICAL PSYCHOLOGY, LEIDEN UNIVERSITY, THE NETHERLANDS

The Field Guide to
BETTER
RESULTS

A companion workbook for *Better Results*

The Field Guide to
BETTER
RESULTS

Evidence-Based
Exercises to Improve
Therapeutic Effectiveness

Edited by

**SCOTT D. MILLER, DARYL CHOW,
SAM MALINS,** and **MARK A. HUBBLE**

Foreword by **BRUCE E. WAMPOLD**

 AMERICAN PSYCHOLOGICAL ASSOCIATION

Published by
American Psychological Association
750 First Street, NE
Washington, DC 20002
https://www.apa.org

Order Department
https://www.apa.org/pubs/books
order@apa.org

In the U.K., Europe, Africa, and the Middle East, copies may be ordered from Eurospan
https://www.eurospanbookstore.com/apa
info@eurospangroup.com

Typeset in Meridien and Ortodoxa by Circle Graphics, Inc., Reisterstown, MD

Printer: Gasch Printing, Odenton, MD
Cover Designer: Mark Karis

Library of Congress Cataloging-in-Publication Data
Names: Miller, Scott D., editor. | Chow, Daryl, editor. | Malins, Sam, editor. |
  Hubble, Mark A., 1951- editor.
Title: The field guide to better results : evidence-based exercises to
  improve therapeutic effectiveness / edited by Scott D. Miller, Daryl Chow,
  Sam Malins, and Mark A. Hubble.
Description: First edition. | Washington, DC : American Psychological
  Association, [2023] | Includes bibliographical references and index.
Identifiers: LCCN 2022054609 (print) | LCCN 2022054610 (ebook) |
  ISBN 9781433837593 (paperback) | ISBN 9781433837609 (ebook)
Subjects: LCSH: Evidence-based psychotherapy. | Psychiatry--Decision making. |
  BISAC: PSYCHOLOGY / Education & Training | PSYCHOLOGY /
  Psychotherapy / Counseling
Classification: LCC RC455.2.E94 F54 2023 (print) | LCC RC455.2.E94 (ebook) |
  DDC 616.89--dc23/eng/20221223
LC record available at https://lccn.loc.gov/2022054609
LC ebook record available at https://lccn.loc.gov/2022054610

https://doi.org/10.1037/0000358-000

Printed in the United States of America

10 9 8 7 6 5 4 3 2 1

CONTENTS

EXPANDED CONTENTS

Introduction: How to Use *The Field Guide to Better Results*   **3**
Scott D. Miller and Mark A. Hubble

Better Results identified the principles and practices associated with using deliberate practice to improve therapeutic effectiveness. As soon as it appeared, readers responded by asking for more—specifically, greater input on how to identify the types of activities most likely to improve results. *The Field Guide* picks up where the previous volume left off by thoroughly reviewing the research on each of the factors responsible for effective therapy as described in the Taxonomy of Deliberate Practice Activities in Psychotherapy (TDPA). Empirically supported principles and exercises are then identified that can be used to develop and fine-tune each therapist's plan for deliberate practice.

1. Identifying Your "What" to Practice   **7**
Scott D. Miller and Mark A. Hubble

Successful deliberate practice depends on creating a plan specifically remedial to an individual's performance deficits. This chapter helps practitioners identify the learning objectives likely to have the greatest leverage in improving their outcomes.

This chapter addresses the second most common question practitioners ask: "After I know what to work on, how am *I* supposed to practice to improve?" It involves mapping performance data onto the factor having the most leverage on outcome, narrowing down potential targets for improvement to a single objective, and breaking the process down into a series of small steps known as a "learning project." Whether you are a "data geek" or "dataphobe," this chapter sets the stage for successful deliberate practice.

Client factors are thought to explain the largest proportion of variance in psychotherapy outcomes. In this chapter, the relevant research linked to change in psychotherapy is reviewed. From this, four evidence-based principles are derived. Seven exercises designed to help therapists develop and refine their abilities for personalizing psychotherapy to the individual client are presented.

It is well established the individual therapist makes a difference for client outcomes. Researchers have gathered information on which aspects of the therapist's personal and professional functioning matter and those that are less relevant. In this chapter, the empirical research in the realm of therapist effects and evidence-based therapist factors is reviewed. Based on the findings, three evidence-based principles and a variety of deliberate practice exercises for enhancing therapist factors in psychotherapy are presented.

The empirical research on relationship factors in psychotherapy is summarized, beginning with a synopsis of relationship factors that do not make a difference in client success. Factors that do make a positive difference are considered next, including the therapeutic alliance (including collaboration and goal consensus), empathy, positive regard and affirmation, therapist congruence and genuineness, the real relationship, emotional expression, and repair of alliance ruptures. From that robust research base, several evidence-based principles are derived, and deliberate practice exercises are recommended.

Client outcome expectation (OE) is the foretelling belief about the likely effectiveness of one's therapy. OE can range on a dimension from less to more hopeful that improvement will occur, and it can shift over time. Thus, OE can be assessed before and repeatedly across therapy to inform treatment planning and therapist responsiveness. This chapter reviews empirical support for the clinical relevance of OE, identifies OE-relevant principles for clinical intervention, offers deliberate practice exercises to help clinicians leverage OE principles, and highlights practice-oriented resources related to OE.

The chapter begins with a brief review of structural factors widely believed to make a difference in the outcome of psychotherapy for which there is little or no evidence: choice of a particular model, fidelity, adherence, competence, universal application of psychological formularies, and unwavering deference to client or therapist preferences. Factors that do make a difference are then considered (e.g., pretreatment preparation or role preparation, problem focus, presence of structure and organization, provision of rationale or credibility, planning for termination), resulting in a transtheoretical metastructure of effective therapeutic structures.

Deliberate practice (DP) is challenging. Most people stop once they have achieved proficiency at a given task. Continuous improvement over the course of one's career requires a sustainable DP plan. Current evidence suggests willpower, motivation, and good intentions are unlikely to be sufficient. To be successful, DP must become a habit. Evidence regarding habit formation is reviewed and distilled into key principles and associated exercises for maintaining engagement in DP over time.

Evidence shows deliberate practice (DP) is more effective than traditional approaches for teaching and training therapists (Barrett-Naylor et al., 2020; Newman et al., 2022; Westra et al., 2021). Still, much remains unknown and subject to revision. This chapter summarizes what is known and offers four concrete suggestions so future work and research remain true to DP's potential for transforming the professional development of psychotherapists.

CONTRIBUTORS

Daryl Chow, PhD, Henry Street Centre, Fremantle, Western Australia
Michael J. Constantino, PhD, Department of Psychological and Brain Sciences, University of Massachusetts Amherst, Amherst, MA, United States
Jaime Delgadillo, PhD, Clinical and Applied Psychology Unit, The University of Sheffield, Sheffield, United Kingdom
Averi N. Gaines, MS, Department of Psychological and Brain Sciences, University of Massachusetts Amherst, Amherst, MA, United States
Erkki Heinonen, PhD, Department of Psychology, University of Oslo, Oslo, Norway
Mark A. Hubble, PhD, International Center for Clinical Excellence, Danbury, CT, United States
Christie P. Karpiak, PhD, Department of Psychology, University of Scranton, Scranton, PA, United States
Sam Malins, DClinPsy, PhD, Institute of Mental Health, University of Nottingham Innovation Park, Nottingham, United Kingdom
Scott D. Miller, PhD, International Center for Clinical Excellence, Chicago, IL, United States
Heather J. Muir, MS, Department of Psychological and Brain Sciences, University of Massachusetts Amherst, Amherst, MA, United States
Helene A. Nissen-Lie, PhD, Department of Psychology, University of Oslo, Oslo, Norway
John C. Norcross, PhD, Department of Psychology, University of Scranton, Scranton, PA, United States
Nicholas Oleen-Junk, PhD, Psychology Resources, League City, TX, United States

Kimberly Ouimette, BS, Department of Psychological and Brain Sciences, University of Massachusetts Amherst, Amherst, MA, United States

Jesse Owen, PhD, Department of Counseling Psychology, University of Denver; Sondermind: OrgVitals: Celesthealth: Lifelong, Denver, CO, United States

Joshua K. Swift, PhD, Department of Psychology, Idaho State University, Pocatello, ID, United States

Bruce E. Wampold, PhD, Department of Counseling Psychology, University of Wisconsin–Madison, Madison, WI, United States

Noah Yulish, PhD, The Willow Center for Integrative Health, Chicago, IL, United States

FOREWORD

So much in our lives rapidly changes. Over 40 years ago, when I started my career studying psychotherapy and training therapists, if I wanted to reach someone, I either mailed a letter or called on a phone tethered to a wall. If I needed to find an article, I physically went to the library and looked through "the stacks." To do a statistical analysis for a study, I punched data onto IBM cards, submitted the deck to the computer center on campus, and returned the next morning to receive the results (that is if I didn't mistake a colon for a semicolon). No personal computers, ethernet, internet, wireless networks, streaming music, and so on . . . and so on.

It is an understatement. Much has changed in these 40-plus years—that is, except how we train therapists and how therapists work to get better over their careers. Sure, we have new therapy models—growing in number every year. However, then, as now, we teach trainees basic therapy skills and some treatment models, then we have them see clients in a practicum. Under the best of circumstances, their work is observed, and supervision is provided. Unfortunately, the process typically focuses on the client and the client's diagnosis; if feedback is provided, it is usually quite general and not focused on particular therapy skills. After that? More clients and more supervision. Then, graduation. More of the same follows, with newly minted therapists documenting hours (not their skills) and passing an examination. After licensing, more lectures, reading, and new models. In some countries, continued supervision is required but, again, rarely focused on providing feedback on specific skills. Is it any wonder therapists do not improve over the course of their careers? Indeed, in terms of outcome, practicing therapists are, on average, equivalent to trainees (yes, we confidently supervise them, believing our years of experience make us experts!).

Attention readers: We need something different. Something based on the science of expertise. Something that will actually lead to better results. Anders Ericsson, who recently passed away, spent his career as a professor of psychology studying expertise. His essential conclusion was that to improve in any domain, individuals must deliberately practice the skills needed for successful performance. Fortunately for the field, Scott Miller and Daryl Chow became aware of Anders's work and enlisted him to collaborate in applying deliberate practice to our profession. This is revolutionary—finally, a scientific-based means to improve psychotherapy outcomes by having therapists advance their skill level.

The Field Guide to Better Results: Evidence-Based Exercises to Improve Therapeutic Effectiveness, edited by Scott D. Miller, Daryl Chow, Sam Malins, and Mark A. Hubble, is an extension of *Better Results: Using Deliberate Practice to Improve Therapeutic Effectiveness* (Miller et al., 2020), which provided readers with the first detailed application of deliberate practice to psychotherapy. In any domain, before one can practice deliberately, the skills needed for successful performance must be identified. Thankfully, this work has been done. The factors that characterize effective therapists are now known. In each chapter of *The Field Guide to Better Results*, the authors (all experts on a particular factor) review decades of research, extracting accessible, essential evidence-based principles, and then offer concrete exercises for skill development.

Improving performance in any domain is difficult, and using deliberate practice to enhance outcomes involves focused effort. As anyone who has dieted knows, we only stick to a program if it works and the work toward the goal is realistic and engaging. Fortunately, *The Field Guide to Better Results* is not only pragmatic but also engaging.

The quality of mental health care depends on effective therapists. We have a duty to our clients and society to provide the most effective services we can. The best way to do this is to deliberately practice the factors responsible for therapeutic change—the goal being for every practitioner to improve continuously.

—*Bruce E. Wampold, PhD*
Professor Emeritus, University of Wisconsin–Madison
and Skillsetter.com

REFERENCE

Miller, S. D., Hubble, M. A., & Chow, D. (2020). *Better results: Using deliberate practice to improve therapeutic effectiveness*. American Psychological Association. https://doi.org/10.1037/0000191-000

A PERSONAL PREFACE AND DEDICATION

Slightly more than 20 years ago, my colleagues and I were struggling with a puzzle. At that time, two tools we had created for monitoring the process and outcome of mental health care were in wide use around the world. The data being generated were providing an intriguing glimpse into real-world clinical practice. Therapists, that evidence clearly showed, were effective—returning outcomes on par with those obtained in tightly controlled randomized clinical trials. Such news was both inspiring and reassuring, especially because it contrasted so sharply with the field's insatiable desire for the "new and improved." Here was a clear and definitive answer. We did good work. Period.

Equally interesting, but inexplicable at the time, were results showing some clinicians were *more* helpful than others—and the difference in effect was far from small. Compared with their more average counterparts, top performers had a much bigger impact on the well-being and functioning of their clients, leading more of them to recovery and doing so in a shorter period. They also appeared to have a knack for helping the most difficult and challenging clients, who, when seen by other therapists, failed to benefit despite many visits.

To be sure, we were not the first group of researchers to find therapists varied in effectiveness. Indeed, published accounts dated back decades. None, however, offered much in the way of explanation for the differences. One exception was a 1974 study of two clinicians, one highly effective "supershrink," the other, based on their comparatively poor results, deemed a "pseudoshrink" (Ricks, 1974). Appearing, as it did, in the pages of an obscure and little-read professional book, this groundbreaking investigation received little subsequent attention. Sadly, the author's promised replication with a larger sample never happened.

With little or no effort, most of us can name specific people across a wide range of human endeavors—art, music, medicine, sports, chess—who have or continue to perform at a *measurably* superior level. The care each of us would put into deciding which mental health professional to recommend for a friend or loved one strongly suggests we believe similar differences exist between providers.

Our idea was simple: Identify the traits, behaviors, training, and practice patterns of highly effective therapists so that the rest of us could emulate their work. Alas, extensive interviews, even watching recordings, provided little insight into what they were doing. As a group, they hewed to no particular theoretical orientation or demographic (e.g., age, gender, years of experience, amount of training, professional degree), and often their work was not especially inspiring to watch. Frankly, much of it was boring, including a mixture of advice-giving, long stretches of inactivity, and trite observations and interpretations. Regarding the process, it could be overly regimented if not controlling, while at others, freewheeling and disorganized.

After much effort, we were forced to face facts. If the best clinicians shared some characteristic or work pattern, we could not see it. For my own part, I was beginning to believe the differences between therapists were simply random. After all, our data set, while large, did not extend very far back in time. Perhaps, as most standard investment disclaimers go, "past performance was no guarantee of future performance." Indeed, maybe it was best to think of a therapist's outcomes like a stock, rising and falling depending on a host of factors not always related to actual ability or accomplishment. The implication, if true, meant nothing could be learned from studying highly effective therapists. They were a mirage—something everyone believed in, even saw, but in reality, did not exist.

The project was shelved following an email exchange with an internationally known colleague and fellow researcher. "The whole idea of 'supershrinks,'" this person asserted, "is burdensome to the hardworking, underpaid, underfunded, and frankly overwhelmed professionals already at significant risk for burning out. Being 'good enough' has to be good enough." And there, our research would have remained had it not been for a chance event.

As shared in our article titled "Supershrinks: What's the Secret of Their Success?" (Miller et al., 2007), I was on a flight home following a training in Europe. Weary from the road and stuck in a middle seat, I gladly took a periodical offered by a passing flight attendant. The magazine, *Fortune*, was new to me. After a quick glance, my attention was immediately drawn to an article titled "What It Takes to be Great" (Colvin, 2006). It showcased the research of Swedish psychologist K. Anders Ericsson, widely regarded as *the* "expert on expertise." He knew why some excelled and others never moved beyond mere proficiency. He had spent his entire career investigating what he termed "deliberate practice" (DP).

I had never heard of him. Once home, however, I made sure to learn as much as I could. Then, I called him. I had been doing that for years—going directly to the source—whenever I had a question or wanted to know more. As an undergraduate, I even had an extended correspondence with B. F. Skinner, first reaching out to him for help with a class assignment.

"Maybe you can educate me a bit about your field," Ericsson said after exchanging the usual pleasantries. Hard to believe, but no mental health professional had ever contacted him. He was surprised to learn how little consensus existed among experts and researchers about what mattered most for success in psychotherapy. With so much disagreement, he observed, "Basically, it's likely individual practitioners will find it difficult to improve." I had to keep myself from laughing out loud. As an outsider to our field, he had no idea how on point he was—later studies would show the outcome of psychotherapy had not improved over the decades, and individual practitioner outcomes actually decline with experience (Germer et al., 2022; Goldberg et al., 2016)!

At the end of our initial contact, he suggested a slew of articles we could read to get up to speed on the subject. More, he expressed a willingness to serve as an advisor should we want to research the application of DP in our profession. In the years that followed, Anders became a trusted friend and consultant, offering encouragement, advice, and critical input on our work and writing. With his inspiration and guidance, we published research in peer-reviewed journals and articles in popular periodicals, documenting the role DP played in the development of highly effective therapists.

Through the application of his ideas, we learned, in contrast to what I initially believed, therapists *were* consistent in their performance—be it good, middling, or bad—and that continuously working to improve one's outcomes did not give rise to burnout but actually prevented it. Later, hoping to add rigor to what remained poor and even contradictory definitions in the empirical literature, we developed a set of criteria by which bona fide instances of DP, therapy-related or not, could be determined—a list successfully used to rebut a study that claimed to show it was far less impactful than Ericsson and his colleagues claimed. Our meta-analysis found

> a relatively large correlation between DP and improved performance compared to other associations considered critical (e.g., the correlations of smoking, obesity, and excessive drinking with mortality). More . . . the magnitude of the relationship is even greater when studies are limited in the analysis to bona fide instances of DP. (Miller et al., 2018, p. 7)

In May 2020, *Better Results: Using Deliberate Practice to Improve Therapeutic Effectiveness* (Miller et al., 2020) was published. It was the culmination of nearly 2 decades of work, thinking, and research. Always encouraging, Ericsson wrote in the foreword, "Its publication heralds . . . a major change in the conception and implementation of training . . . and change in the methods used to ensure continued refinement of . . . therapists' performance through their entire careers" (Miller et al., 2020, p. xiv). For my part, it felt as though we were just getting started. We had the "picture on the box" to guide us and the border and some of the more obvious clusters assembled, but the puzzle was far from complete.

One month after the publication of our book, I interviewed Dr. Ericsson for my blog (Miller, 2020). By this time, my colleagues and I were already developing plans for what would eventually become *The Field Guide to Better Results*. Dr. Ericsson was as stimulating and encouraging as ever. It turns out, after a lifetime of presentations, publications, and interviews, this would be his last. Days following our conversation, Anders died. It was a deep and unexpected personal and professional loss. I miss his accessibility, openness, deep curiosity, and singular focus and hope he would be proud of this volume.

Ending this dedication, I recall his parting words when we last spoke about deliberate practice: "When I talk to people who are very successful . . . they have this daily routine, so they don't really have to ask themselves, 'Do I really *feel* like doing this today?' No! They just start doing it."

—*Scott D. Miller*

REFERENCES

Colvin, G. (2006, October 30). What it takes to be great. *Fortune, 154*(9), 88–96.

Germer, S., Weyrich, V., Bräscher, A.-K., & Witthöft, M. (2022). Does practice really make perfect? A longitudinal analysis of the relationship between therapist experience and therapy outcome. *Journal of Counseling Psychology, 69*(5), 745–754. https://doi.org/10.1037/cou0000608

Goldberg, S. B., Rousmaniere, T., Miller, S. D., Whipple, J., Nielsen, S. L., Hoyt, W. T., & Wampold, B. E. (2016). Do psychotherapists improve with time and experience? A longitudinal analysis of outcomes in a clinical setting. *Journal of Counseling Psychology, 63*(1), 1–11. https://doi.org/10.1037/cou0000131

Miller, S. D. (2020, June 22). *The expert on expertise: An interview with K. Anders Ericsson* [Video]. YouTube. https://www.youtube.com/watch?v=8WARK0aNX88&t=7s

Miller, S. D., Chow, D., Wampold, B., Hubble, M. A., Del Re, A. C., Maeschalck, C., & Bargmann, S. (2018). To be or not to be (an expert)? Revisiting the role of deliberate practice in improving performance. *High Ability Studies, 31*(1), 5–15. https://doi.org/10.1080/13598139.2018.1519410

Miller, S. D., Hubble, M. A., & Chow, D. (2020). *Better results: Using deliberate practice to improve therapeutic effectiveness.* American Psychological Association. https://doi.org/10.1037/0000191-000

Miller, S. D., Hubble, M. A., & Duncan, B. L. (2007, November/December). Supershrinks: Learning from the field's most effective practitioners. *The Psychotherapy Networker, 31*(6), 26–35, 56.

Ricks, D. F. (1974). Supershrink: Methods of a therapist judged successful on the basis of adult outcomes of adolescent patients. In D. F. Ricks & M. Roff (Eds.), *Life history research in psychopathology* (pp. 275–297). University of Minnesota Press.

The Field Guide to
BETTER RESULTS

Introduction

How to Use The Field Guide to Better Results

Scott D. Miller and Mark A. Hubble

You can't use an old map to explore a new world.

—ALBERT EINSTEIN

Welcome to *The Field Guide to Better Results* (*FG*). Books in this genre number in the thousands. A quick search on the internet reveals field guides can be purchased on almost any topic—from ants to zebras, moths to mushrooms, ocean floors to mountain tops, dinosaurs to UFOs and the extraterrestrials who pilot them. Using a combination of short summaries, illustrations, charts, and advice, their specific purpose is to help the user quickly and efficiently identify, locate, and distinguish key characteristics defining the subject of interest—in this instance, the first field guide ever published on using deliberate practice (DP) to improve therapist effectiveness.

The *FG* is the follow-up to *Better Results* (*BR*; Miller et al., 2020). It is best seen as a companion volume, the need for which became evident long before the first work was completed. Although applied across a variety of performance domains (e.g., chess, music, medicine, athletics), DP is a relatively new topic in psychotherapy (Miller & Hubble, 2011; Miller et al., 2007). Conflicting viewpoints regarding its nature and use are already on the rise (Rousmaniere, 2016, 2019). And, in truth, despite the detailed principles and practices described in *BR*, much of the framework provided required further investigation and exposition based on emerging science. In addition, the practitioners we encountered who were trying to apply DP to their professional development wanted

https://doi.org/10.1037/0000358-001
The Field Guide to Better Results: Evidence-Based Exercises to Improve Therapeutic Effectiveness,
S. D. Miller, D. Chow, S. Malins, and M. A. Hubble (Editors)

more—in particular, explicit guidance in a readily accessible format about what to practice deliberately and how.

While reviewing the galley proofs of *BR*, mindful of the work left to be done, we began reaching out to researchers known for their expertise on the factors responsible for the effectiveness of psychotherapy (e.g., client, therapist, relationship, hope and expectancy, structure). Each was invited to (a) review the latest empirical literature on a specific factor, (b) distill evidence-based principles for empowering it, and last, (c) create exercises practitioners could immediately perform to strengthen the operation of the principles in their clinical work. Without exception, all agreed to contribute.

In Chapter 3, Joshua K. Swift, Jesse Owen, and Scott D. Miller focus on the contribution to outcome made by the client. Research shows who they are; what qualities, traits, and experiences they bring to therapy; and what influences in their life outside of treatment have the largest effect on results. In Chapter 4, Helen A. Nissen-Lie, Erkki Heinonen, and Jaime Delgadillo direct their attention to what pioneering researcher Sol Garfield (1997) once called "the neglected variable" in psychotherapy: the therapist. Turns out, *who* does the therapy is of critical importance, far more so than any method or approach. John C. Norcross and Christie P. Karpiak, in Chapter 5, delineate the characteristics of productive helping relationships, adding the nuance and detail necessary to enable practitioners to customize their connection to each client. Helping clinicians understand the role of hope and expectancy and how beliefs in the effectiveness of a given course of mental health care can be supported and strengthened is the subject of Chapter 6 by Michael J. Constantino, Heather J. Muir, Averi N. Gaines, and Kimberly Ouimette. Finally, in Chapter 7, Nicholas Oleen-Junk and Noah Yulish address the last of the factors responsible for the effectiveness: structure. Structure includes the therapeutic rationale, associated techniques and rituals, the timing of interventions, and the treatment context or setting. Regardless of a clinician's preferred way of working, this chapter shows how to organize and execute care for maximum benefit.

Beyond the identification of evidence-based principles and specific exercises, some clinicians reported wanting more help than was provided in *BR* for getting started and sustaining their DP efforts. Expressed, too, was an interest in how to narrow down potential professional development targets to the single learning objective, which, when reached, would yield the greatest return on investment. In the first chapter, Scott D. Miller and Mark A. Hubble offer insight and advice for practitioners who, despite being interested in DP, have yet to move past the "this-is-a-good-idea" phase. Later in the book, in Chapter 8, Sam Malins, Scott D. Miller, Mark A. Hubble, and Daryl Chow address what to do when one's implementation is marked by fits and starts. Finally, in the second chapter, Daryl Chow, Scott D. Miller, and Mark A. Hubble offer solutions for those feeling overwhelmed in their attempt to select the best learning objective from among the many possibilities. As first introduced in *BR*, the Taxonomy of Deliberate Practice Activities in Psychotherapy (Chow & Miller, 2022) plays a key role in helping practitioners develop an individualized, step-by-step professional development plan (a revised and updated version can be found in Appendix A).

Unlike *BR*, the *FG* is not designed to be read from cover to cover. Instead, it's best thought of as a reference work, a resource to consult whenever a specific question, decision point, or challenge arises in one's application of DP. Like any field guide, the section that has the most relevance depends on where the person is and what they need to know or be able to do *now*.

If you are ready to get going with the *FG*, consult the map in Figure 1. It will help identify "where you are" in your implementation of DP and point you to the next step. For convenience and to help you stay on track, key decision points selected from the map are included at the beginning and end of each chapter.

FIGURE 1. The *Field Guide* Map

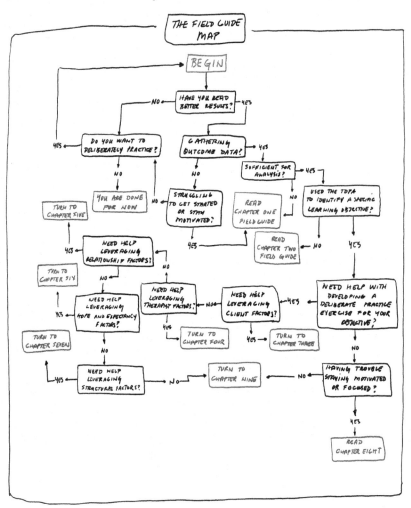

REFERENCES

Chow, D., & Miller, S. D. (2022). *Taxonomy of Deliberate Practice Activities in Psychotherapy—Therapist Version* (Version 6). International Center for Clinical Excellence.

Garfield, S. L. (1997). The therapist as a neglected variable in psychotherapy research. *Clinical Psychology: Science and Practice, 4*(1), 40–43. https://doi.org/10.1111/j.1468-2850.1997.tb00097.x

Miller, S. D., & Hubble, M. (2011). The road to mastery. *Psychotherapy Networker, 35*(3).

Miller, S. D., Hubble, M., & Chow, D. (2020). *Better results: Using deliberate practice to improve therapeutic effectiveness.* American Psychological Association. https://doi.org/10.1037/0000191-000

Miller, S. D., Hubble, M. A., & Duncan, B. L. (2007). Supershrinks: What's the secret of their success? *Psychotherapy Networker, 31*(6).

Rousmanicre, T. (2016). *Deliberate practice for psychotherapists: A guide to improving clinical effectiveness.* Routledge. https://doi.org/10.4324/9781315472256

Rousmaniere, T. G. (2019). *Mastering the inner skills of psychotherapy: A deliberate practice handbook.* Gold Lantern Books.

1

Identifying Your "What" to Practice

Scott D. Miller and Mark A. Hubble

The illiterate of the 21st century will not be those who cannot read and write, but those who cannot learn, unlearn, and relearn.

—ALVIN TOFFLER

DECISION POINT

Begin here if you have read the book *Better Results* and

- have not started gathering outcome data or are experiencing difficulty getting started or maintaining the motivation to measure your performance *or*

- are measuring your performance but have not collected sufficient data to establish a reliable, evidence-based profile of your therapeutic effectiveness.

No question. Practitioners are a motivated bunch. They want to improve. They value learning. They are committed to professional development. In the largest, most comprehensive survey conducted to date, 86% of clinicians reported being "highly motivated" to transcend their current level of performance (Orlinsky & Rønnestad, 2005).

https://doi.org/10.1037/0000358-002
The Field Guide to Better Results: Evidence-Based Exercises to Improve Therapeutic Effectiveness,
S. D. Miller, D. Chow, S. Malins, and M. A. Hubble (Editors)

It starts early. Admission to graduate programs is highly competitive, with ratios of 300 applicants to 8 positions being commonplace (Info Learners, 2022). Once in, the work continues, even intensifies: classes, practica, exams, theses, and dissertations. "Curriculum creep" has come to define graduate education, with the number of required hours increasing 25% over the last 30 years (Caldwell, 2015). Thousands of hours of supervision follow—a practice most clinicians deem critical to their professional development and of help throughout their careers. Close behind is personal therapy. Most go (Bike et al., 2009; Norcross, 2005). And not just for a single course but returning time and again. By the way, those who do not report the *lowest* experience of "felt progress" and *highest* career "regress and stasis" (Orlinsky & Rønnestad, 2005, p. 121).

There is more. Graduate education does not end with graduate school. Though required for licensure, practitioners enthusiastically pursue continuing education. They do so to maintain and update their knowledge and skills (Neimeyer et al., 2009; Neimeyer & Taylor, 2011). In the United States, psychologists—the authors conservatively estimate[1]—spend $38 million per year on such activities. This amount excludes the costs of travel, lodging, food, supplementary learning materials (e.g., books, videos), and for some, lost revenue.

Given clinicians' dedication to lifelong learning, it should come as no surprise the arrival of deliberate practice (DP) on the professional scene has attracted considerable interest. Before 2007, the term had never been heard, much less used in the context of psychotherapy research or training. That year, Miller, Hubble, and Duncan introduced the field to the work of Swedish psychologist K. Anders Ericsson. In numerous studies conducted over 3 decades, he and other researchers had documented how DP, regardless of domain (e.g., sports, music, medicine, chess, teaching), was responsible for superior performance. On review of this work, Miller et al. (2007) proposed DP provided an answer to a question that had long eluded the field—one that pioneering outcome researcher Michael Lambert only a few years earlier had characterized as "a mystery." To wit, why are some therapists *consistently* and *significantly* more effective than others?

When subsequent research confirmed the most effective therapists devote a larger amount of time to DP than others (Chow et al., 2015), practitioners—always hungry for guidance and direction—responded, "Just tell us how to do it and what to practice, and we'll do it." As commendable as this openness and willingness to learn is, unfortunately, if given what they ask for, no doubt, the gains desired will never be realized.

That last sentence bears rereading.

Turns out, the promise of DP is in danger of being undermined. Historically, the mental health professions have never suffered from a shortage of experts ready and willing to tell practitioners what to do to be effective (Hubble et al., 1999). The premise has, and continues to be, practice this method or that

---

[1]The estimate was derived by multiplying the number of licensed psychologists in the United States by the hours of continuing education required to maintain their licensure and the average cost of each continuing education hour as of 2021.

technique until proficiency is reached, and professional growth is assured. Not surprisingly, in the 15 short years since DP was first introduced to psychotherapy, a series of books have appeared applying the term to mastering specific treatment models (e.g., cognitive behavior therapy, emotion-focused therapy), even promising certification as a therapist or coach in the process. Though few in number at present, studies within the field have followed suit, frequently mistaking repetition and rehearsal for *deliberate* practice (Chow et al., 2022). *They are not the same.* The fallacy of this approach, as detailed in Chapter 2 of *Better Results* (*BR*; Miller, Hubble, & Chow, 2020), is research evidence convincingly demonstrates training in specific theories and their associated techniques contribute little, if anything, to outcome.

So, what should practitioners do instead?

Before embarking on a course of professional development, each must answer the question "What do *I* need to target to improve my particular results?" Although it may sound bold, failing to provide a detailed, evidence-based, and therapist-specific answer to this question all but guarantees (a) clinician effectiveness will remain flat, as has been seen in the field for the past 40 years or (b) decline, as studies of individual therapist outcomes show happens, regardless of the amount of time, money, and energy invested in learning something new (Germer et al., 2022; Goldberg et al., 2016; Prochaska et al., 2020; Wampold & Imel, 2015). For all that, the demands of daily clinical work often make the promise of "do this and you'll help more people" difficult to resist.

PRINCIPLES FOR IDENTIFYING YOUR WHAT

In what follows, four evidence-based principles are identified and described, each aimed at helping practitioners prepare for effective DP. The principles are, in turn, operationalized in a set of exercises found at the end of the chapter.

Principle 1: Avoid the Athenian Trap

Clearly, K. Anders Ericsson and colleagues were not thinking of how to pitch their ideas to the masses when, in their original 1993 article on expertise published in the *American Psychologist*, they wrote, "In contrast to play, . . . deliberate practice . . . is not inherently enjoyable, [and] generates no immediate . . . rewards" (p. 368). Both experience and subsequent research confirm the accuracy of their observations (Miller, Madsen, & Hubble, 2020).

Plainly put, DP is hard work. Once a modicum of proficiency has been achieved in a particular performance domain, interest in pushing oneself typically wanes (Ericsson & Pool, 2016). Moreover, as confidence increases—generally far outstripping actual, measured ability—most turn their attention to something more stimulating. It is not solely a question of motivation or willpower. The brain, hardwired for novelty, naturally selects and rewards the "new and different" (Bunzeck & Düzel, 2006).

The allure of the unfamiliar is as old as recorded history. Consider: In the Biblical book of Acts, the citizens of Athens are described as "spend[ing] their time doing nothing but talking about and listening to the latest ideas" (17:21). So pervasive was this behavior, even the celebrated Greek historian and general, Thucydides (460–400 BCE), described the Athenian people as routinely "deceived with the novelty of speech" (Barnes, 1981).

When it comes to professional development, it is as though therapists live in a modern-day version of Athens. Talk of fresh, exciting discoveries, cutting-edge research, and improved theories and methods is constant and inescapable, all breathlessly reported. The underlying promise? The "state-of-the-art" is one workshop or certification away.

To have any chance of being successful in using DP to improve therapeutic effectiveness, therapists will need to immunize themselves against the "Athenian trap." Isolation, boredom, frustration, uncertainty, comparing oneself with others (and failing in the comparison), and enduring extended periods of little or no apparent progress are part of the process. They are also potent triggers. In all likelihood, others exist, varying from one person to the next.

At the end of this chapter, you will find an exercise designed to improve your chances of both mobilizing and maintaining the motivation required for DP.

Principle 2: Finding Your What

The idea that improvement depends on practice is hardly new. References to enhancing a person's skills or abilities through focused concentration and effort date back more than 2 millennia (Amirault & Branson, 2006; Ericsson, 2006b). Though DP includes the word *practice*, it is altogether different. The highly individualized nature of the process separates it from what practice is most commonly considered to be. Truly, the goal of DP is neither proficiency nor mastery. Rather, it is all about continuously reaching for objectives that lie just beyond one's current ability. Accomplishing this task relies on a data-derived identification of "what" specifically each individual needs to target to improve their performance. As emphasized in *BR*, one must begin with identifying the "what" before the "how" (see Miller et al., 2020, pp. 43–47).

Over the last 2 decades, several outcome measurement systems have been developed, tested, and utilized in real-world clinical settings (Miller, Hubble, & Chow, 2020). Most include detailed metrics which enable the clinician-user to develop an evidence-based profile of their work—what, where, and with whom they excel and, more important, where they fall short or could make improvements. Detailed information was provided about one of the most widely used—The Partners for Change Outcome Management System—in *BR* (Miller, Hubble, & Chow, 2020, pp. 51–57).

While the technological capacity to identify one's "growth edge" is now widely available, some therapists struggle to begin using measures or, once started, employ them consistently in their work. To be frank, ongoing, real-time assessment of clinical performance using standardized scales is new to the profession—so much so most have never heard of it, much less received any formal training in the process (Hatfield & Ogles, 2007; Madsen et al., 2021). As is true with almost every endeavor, a learning curve exists. In the case of the two instruments described in *BR*, their simplicity belies the difficulty research shows clinicians encounter when implementing them in their daily work (Brattland et al., 2018). Another consideration—beyond lack of knowledge, training, or experience—is the attitude of the clinician. Not surprisingly, the evidence documents some are more open to the performance feedback measurement provides (de Jong et al., 2012).

If the foregoing were not enough, therapists need to be prepared; the feedback received can be highly disruptive. No, it *is* highly disruptive. No, it *must be* highly disruptive to qualify as DP. In a series of intriguing studies, Chow and colleagues (Chow et al., 2022; Miller et al., 2015) found engaging in DP delivered a blow to therapist confidence. The good news is the reduction in self-assurance enabled therapists first to consider and then make changes in their behavior, thereby resulting in measured improvements in performance. Such findings are entirely consistent with evidence from other investigations demonstrating therapists higher on professional self-doubt and humility establish stronger therapeutic relationships and achieve better outcomes (Nissen-Lie et al., 2010; Nissen-Lie & Rønnestad, 2016; Tao et al., 2015; see also Chapter 4, this volume).

As a case in point, take the example of Brooke Mathewes, an accomplished and well-regarded psychotherapist working in the United States. For all her success in the profession, the passion of her life is horses. As a child, she dreamed of being a cowgirl, decorating her bedroom with toy horses, horse paintings, and books about horses. The curtains were even hung with wrought-iron horseshoes.

Talk with Brooke and, in short order, the conversation inevitably turns to the time she spends at McGinnis Meadows Ranch. There, she's had the privilege of being mentored by Shayne, one of the world's most celebrated "horse whisperers"—a person with an uncanny, almost magical ability to engage and heal animals with a history of mistreatment, if not outright abuse.

From the outset, Brooke was a highly motivated student. Her goal? Replicate her mentor's success. Toward that end, she spent hours watching him work, observing his every move: his voice, how he walked, the movement of his hands, even the angle of his feet in the stirrups. Contributing to her mounting frustration, he would often say, "Watch closely now. If you blink, you'll miss it."

Brooke recalls, "I must have been blinking a lot."

Continuing, "Early on, my confidence was badly shaken. I'd ridden for years, spent uncountable hours with horses, but couldn't match, or see what Shayne was doing. Even when he gave me explicit directions, I still couldn't make it work. That's when my thoughts would turn harsh. '*I'm never going to get this. Cowgirl-shmowgirl. I'm just not good enough.*'" Many times, Brooke was tempted to give up. Pack up her tack, saddle, and boots and go back to riding at the stable near her home.

Pausing, she then shares, "In time, and with Shayne's ongoing encouragement and coaching, I became better at finding my 'sweet spot of discomfort,' actively seeking out experiences that pushed me beyond what I could do at the moment, but not so far as to risk being crushed whenever I fell short of the mark." How Brooke achieved this balance, ultimately improving her ability to attune to horses *and* transferring her understanding to clinical work, is described in depth in the *Psychotherapy Networker* article "Meet You in McGinnis Meadows" (Mathewes & Miller, 2020). Suffice it to say, the first step is befriending doubt, seeing it as a bridge to learning and not as a referendum on one's performance.

Principle 3: Connecting Your What to the "Right Stuff"

Physicians at Vienna General Hospital had a major problem. In the mid-1840s, women giving birth at this premier facility were dying—at a rate of 25% to 30%. The cause was well-known, accepted medical science dating back to the "father of medicine" himself, Hippocrates (460–370 BCE). Miasma was the culprit. Bad air. Fog, pollution, defilement, and emanations from rotting organic matter. In the words of Roman architect Marcus Vitruvius Pollio (70–15 BCE), it was "mist from marshes . . . blow[ing] toward the town at sunrise . . . waft[ing] into the bodies of inhabitants" (Karamanou et al., 2012, p. 52).

The solution? Eliminate waste. Clean the streets. Urge people to close their doors and windows. Two millennia later, the same explanation held sway. "All smell is disease," asserted the English social reformer, Sir Edwin Chadwick (1800–1890), giving rise to an entire movement aimed at improving public health. And in truth, such strategies were followed by reductions in the spread of certain diseases (e.g., cholera). On the obstetrics ward, however, miasma was not deterred. It remained a killer—a tricky, even cunning one at that.

Enter Ignaz Semmelweis. For him, something about prevailing medical wisdom did not add up. Literally. Midwives working at the same hospital, he observed, had a death rate 6 times lower than the medical staff. Following the death of a colleague who fell ill after puncturing a finger while performing an autopsy, Semmelweis had an epiphany. Contact with corpses was somehow associated with morbidity and mortality. He suggested all contact with patients be preceded and followed by handwashing (Miller, Madsen, & Hubble, 2020). In no time, the mortality rate in the maternity ward plummeted, dropping to the same level as that of midwives. Similar results were obtained when he implemented the same practice in another hospital in Pest, Hungary.

One might expect such a discovery, in addition to bringing about the abandonment of miasma theory, would have earned Semmelweis many honors and awards. It did neither. In fact, his views were rejected by his colleagues and the field alike. Handwashing simply could not compete with bad air, in theory or practice. In 1865, after penning what many consider one of the most important volumes on infectious diseases in history, friends lured him into visiting a mental asylum. Convinced his unrelenting and strident advocacy of handwashing was a sign of mental instability, they forcibly detained him. In a cruel twist of fate, the injuries he sustained in the process became infected, and he died of septicemia 2 weeks later.

Nowadays, of course, the benefits of sanitation are universally accepted. Handwashing, in particular, is considered a "best practice." Indeed, decades of research show it to be the single most effective way to prevent the spread of infections. Science has also discovered why good hygiene works. It kills germs. Such information was not available to Semmelweis or his contemporaries. His was a hunch—one that defied 2,000 years of medical understanding. As sad as it is, what happened is not at all surprising. Unable to connect the declining death rate on the obstetrics ward with the factor responsible for the success of handwashing, his ideas were rejected, and with the benefits of general sanitation efforts elsewhere, belief in miasma continued.

The parallel between the story just shared and contemporary psychotherapy could not be more obvious. Standard interventions such as confronting dysfunctional thoughts, initiating saccadic eye movements, raising emotional awareness, facilitating understanding of internal conflicts, and enhancing communication skills are the miasma "abatement" strategies of our day. Indeed, despite 50 years of theorizing and research, scant evidence exists documenting a causal connection between the use of *any* specific method or technique and treatment outcomes (Wampold & Imel, 2015). Accordingly, making such procedures the primary focus of one's deliberate practice is about as likely to lead to an improvement in therapeutic effectiveness as closing the windows of one's home will stop the spread of disease.

Achieving better results requires connecting an individual's performance objectives to factors that actually have leverage on outcomes. A general review of these empirically established elements can be found in Chapter 11 of *BR* (Miller, Hubble, & Chow, 2020, pp. 115–122). Detailed reviews of the supporting research for each, along with evidence-based principles and exercises, are provided in subsequent chapters of the *Field Guide*—specifically, 3, 4, 5, 6, and 7. In the meantime, recall, in order of influence, the factors include (a) client and extratherapeutic factors, (b) alliance and relationship, (c) therapist effects, (d) hope and expectancy, and (e) structure. More, they form the basis of the Taxonomy of Deliberate Practice Activities in Psychotherapy (TDPA; Chow & Miller, 2022; see Appendix A of this volume)—a tool designed to (a) help align your "what" with the factors likely to exert the greatest impact on performance, (b) design effective DP exercises, and (c) monitor progress of your professional development efforts (Miller, Hubble, & Chow, 2020, pp. 179–192). Unfortunately, experience has shown, if one's theoretical premises and presuppositions are not carefully examined and, if need be, ruthlessly challenged, no amount of time and effort will make a difference.

Refer to the end of this chapter for two exercises that will help you examine your core beliefs, bring how you work into bold relief, and consequently, derive the most benefit from completing the TDPA.

Principle 4: Keep Your Eyes on the Next Step (*Not* the Prize)

The distance between Camp 4 and the summit of K2—the world's second-highest peak—is a mere 2,100 feet. Given an average human stride of 30 inches, that amounts to 840 steps. Based on the numbers alone, it would seem a relatively easy task. And yet, only 377 people have ever succeeded, fewer than have been to outer space! By comparison, climbing Everest is a cakewalk. Despite being taller, 10 times as many have reached the top. Even then, nearly one in five dies trying, a rate that increases 60% when K2 is the objective.

Understanding why people commit massive amounts of time, effort, and resources to such pursuits, even risking their lives, has been the subject of many articles and research studies. Is it the competitive spirit? Natural human curiosity? A desire for fame or notoriety? The pride of achieving a goal few would even consider attempting? Or is it simply as famed British mountaineer George Mallory (who perished on his third attempt at Everest) replied, "Because it's there."

The very same question faces those who would engage in DP: *Why do it?* DP consumes a significant amount of time. Progress often comes in small increments and at a rate that is positively glacial. On top, the typical incentives (e.g., money, status, advancement, validation) are rarely, if ever, commensurate with the investment. That is why, right up to his death, K. Anders Ericsson remained puzzled about what motivated those who choose to engage in DP—calling it the "million-dollar question."

Turns out, as is the case with mountain climbers, the reasons therapists give for continuously pushing the limits of their performance vary. Some feel ethically compelled, duty bound to offer the best to their clients. For others, it is the satisfaction, even joy, that comes with ongoing learning and professional growth.

Setting questions of motivation aside, perhaps the more, if not most important consideration is how to make oneself ready for the sustained effort DP demands. As a rule, determination, no matter how great, will, in time, succumb to poor preparation. The good news is that preparation works in tandem with determination *when* one maintains a singular focus on the next step needed to accomplish a just noticeable difference over what one was able to do before. While the empirical evidence in this area is thin, experience indicates those who are successful relish the achievement of each advance as much as or more than reaching the final, desired outcome (Colvin, 2008). Instead of keeping your eye on the prize, prize each step.

Returning to K2, by the final stage of their ascent, climbers have generally been in transit for months. Even getting to the base of the mountain is an ordeal, requiring 7 or 8 days of difficult trekking over rocky terrain on narrow paths. Then, there are the first three camps, each one at a higher altitude than the last. The terrain is treacherous, the air increasingly thin, generally forcing climbers to stay for days along the way to rest and acclimatize. Many are forced to backtrack multiple times just to "catch their breath"—a process that can take 3 to 4 weeks! Without exception, those who make it to Camp 4 find themselves short of supplies, physically and mentally exhausted, and starved for oxygen. They are also facing the most dangerous part of the climb, the spot responsible for the majority of deaths on K2. It is known as "the bottleneck," and it's not technically difficult, but the house-sized columns of glacial ice bordering the near vertical crevasse (known as *seracs* and *couloir*, respectively) have a tendency to give way unexpectedly. Given the context, each step short of the summit *is* a remarkable accomplishment.

While not putting their lives on the line, therapists do face a bottleneck of sorts. Actually, two. First, unlike the feeling of accomplishment climbers experience on reaching the summit of K2, few, if any, incentives exist for therapists choosing to engage in DP. Beyond the absence of direct financial rewards for superior results—after all, being average pays the same rate—current standards of care do not require clinicians to work at improving their effectiveness. In the *Ethical Principles of Psychologists and Code of Conduct*, for example, the word "effective" does not appear a single time. Rather, practitioners need only "provide services . . . with populations and in areas . . . within the boundaries of their competence, based on their education, training, supervised experience, consultation, study, or professional expertise" (Standard 2.01, Boundaries of Competence, American Psychological Association, 2017, p. 5). Perversely, that means, as Miller, Madsen, and Hubble (2020) pointed out, "a practitioner who competently delivers an unhelpful, even deadly service . . . [is ethically] superior to one who is actually helpful but working beyond" (p. 952) what they are currently capable of doing—the very heart of DP.

The second and far greater challenge for therapists hoping to improve via DP is their current level of effectiveness (see *BR*, pp. 49–58). Evidence from practicing clinicians shows most are remarkably effective, returning outcomes on par with those reported in tightly controlled randomized trials—investigations in which it should be noted study clinicians have many advantages over their real-world counterparts (e.g., access to the best, ongoing training and supervision, lower and less complex caseloads; Minami et al., 2008; Reese et al., 2014; Saxon & Barkham, 2012; Stiles et al., 2008). Said another way, were K2 the objective, the average practitioner would typically be *starting* their DP journey at Camp 4! The remaining steps before their "summit," while not technically difficult, are bound to be the steepest and most slow going. What is more, unlike any prior professional development experiences, the path forward is subject to life circumstances and conditions (e.g., family, job, health, finances, the ease of an established way of working vs. trying something new) that can, without warning, upend the best intentions.

Think of it this way: If you are reading this book, chances are you have finished graduate school and are working in an applied setting. It may be difficult to recall, but at one time, *that* was your objective—to be a full-fledged, working therapist. Of course, doing so was preceded by preschool and kindergarten, the elementary grades, junior and senior high school, and then college. Along the way, you took hundreds of tests and completed an untold number of long-forgotten reading and homework assignments.

With effort and focus, you can likely remember the sense of pride you felt on passing the final exam for a challenging undergraduate course, despite having many more to complete before graduating. How about the sense of relief you experienced when you finished collecting data for your thesis or dissertation? More than likely, you did so even though crunching the numbers, writing up the results, and defending your project before your faculty committee remained. And what about passing the licensing exam? We are sure you will agree doing so was a significant achievement, although finding a job, building a practice, and establishing yourself in the profession was yet to be realized.

The point? Though your final objective may still be before you, it need not detract from the satisfaction you experience with each step. Indeed, reaching your summit will require as much. Otherwise, we run the risk of remaining in the demotivating state of continuous presuccess failure (Adams, 2013).

SUMMARY

Effective DP begins with identifying "what" you specifically need to target to improve your effectiveness. Because the pattern of performance strengths and weaknesses is different for each clinician, no prepackaged, one-size-applied-to-all set of skills or exercises will work. Therapists hoping to achieve better results do well to avoid anyone promising otherwise (Principle 1: Avoid the Athenian Trap). Instead, the process begins with each establishing an evidence-based profile of their work, using a valid and reliable set of measurement tools to identify what they do well and where they could do better (Principle 2: Finding Your What). To ensure that what we practice makes a difference, it must then be connected to factors that actually have leverage on outcome (Principle 3: Connecting Your What to the Right Stuff). Research shows most of what is popularly believed to be responsible for the efficacy of psychotherapy contributes little or nothing to the outcome (e.g., treatment models and techniques, professional and postgraduate training, supervision). Now in its sixth revision, the TDPA is specifically designed to help connect individual practitioner performance improvement efforts to what really makes a difference. The next chapter provides tips for maximizing the utility of the tool based on feedback from users gathered since its publication in *BR*. Chief among the suggestions is helping develop the single DP objective necessary to accomplish a just noticeable difference in what one was able to do before (Principle 4: Keep Your Eyes on the Next Step).

EXERCISES FOR IDENTIFYING YOUR WHAT

In what follows, the principles identified in the previous section are linked to specific DP exercises. While several may strike you as compelling or interesting, avoid the temptation to "get to work." Instead, read through them all, choosing those specifically tied to your current professional development objectives.

Principle 1: Avoid the Athenian Trap

The isolation, boredom, frustration, uncertainty, and extended periods of little or no apparent progress can disrupt the DP efforts of even the most dedicated. Given that the specifics will be different for each individual, it can be helpful to take the time to identify your triggers—what might tempt you from the focus required for success. So, whether using paper and pencil or an electronic device, list yours, being as detailed and specific as possible.

To help you get started, consider the following questions:

- *What specifically could tempt you to forgo DP in favor of less demanding, more enjoyable, but ineffective professional development activities?*

- *What role, if any, do people, places, emotional states, prior training, clinical beliefs, experiences, and so forth play in thwarting the focused, ongoing effort and concentration required for DP?*

Once you have identified your specific triggers,

- *Recall a time in the past when you were tempted to stray but stayed on course. Include experiences outside the professional realm (e.g., learning a second language or to play a musical instrument).*

- *What role, if any, did people, places, emotional states, personal beliefs and experiences, and so forth play in supporting and sustaining your commitment to success?*

- *How will you incorporate and use the natural human predisposition for novelty into your DP plan?*

Finish by providing answers to the following questions:

- *On a scale from 0 to 10, where 0 denotes* none *and 10* absolute certainty, *rate your current level of confidence in your ability to manage triggers.*

- *Identify a circumstance that you might encounter that would lower your current rating.*

- *Imagine what it would take to* raise *your rating by a single point.*

Principle 2: Finding Your What

Introducing measurement into one's clinical performance can be highly disruptive; the process of administering scales and reviewing the results may undermine confidence. Fortunately, the evidence indicates disruptions that result in reductions in self-assurance can enable therapists to accept and make needed changes in how they work, thereby resulting in stronger therapeutic relationships and better outcomes.

The following exercise is designed to help you embrace your doubt, seeing it as a bridge to learning and not as a referendum on your performance. Take the time necessary to reflect on and respond to the following questions:

- *Identify several circumstances—whether as a clinician or in your personal life—when you felt doubt about your knowledge, skills, or ability to succeed.*

- *Contrast the times when you embraced the doubt necessary for change or surrendered to it and gave up. Recall in as much detail as possible the context (i.e., where you were, who you were with, your thoughts, feelings, and actions).*

- *Imagine what feelings, thoughts, and behaviors will arise for you while "inhabiting" your sweet spot of discomfort. How will you stay focused on what you are learning versus giving in to a sense of incompetence and feelings of shame that so often accompany failed attempts?*

Principle 3: Connecting Your What to the Right Stuff

Getting to the Source of Your Success (Part 1)

Effective DP requires connecting an individual's performance objective to factors that have leverage on outcomes. As noted earlier and reviewed in detail in Chapter 2, the TDPA is specifically designed to help align our professional development efforts with what matters most for improving our results.

There is more. Early on in *BR*, we recommended creating a schematic or blueprint for how you do therapy sufficiently detailed enough that another practitioner could understand and replicate it—literally, "step into your shoes" and work how you work (Miller, Hubble, & Chow, 2020, p. 29). The purpose of the exercise was to make it possible for clinicians to pinpoint where in their work they could intervene once their "what" had been identified. To illustrate, did the "what" occur throughout the course of therapy or at certain points (i.e., beginning, middle, or end)? Was it related to one's theoretical premises (e.g., a point of view that undermined the formation and maintenance of the therapeutic relationship)? Was it linked to the overall plan of action (e.g., strategies and objectives that failed to elicit the client's active participation)? Or finally, was the "what" connected to one's use of a particular technique or its execution?

Feedback received following the publication of *BR* revealed this exercise to be among the most difficult in the volume to complete. Many readers reported having difficulty knowing where to begin (e.g., start with their preferred theory, what they typically do in a first session, describing the temporal sequence of their work). Others, when prompted to describe their work as a series of "if–then" propositions (e.g., IF the client presents as highly reactive, THEN I adopt a more flexible, nondirective stance; IF the client reports depression at the first visit, THEN I assign a "thought log" as homework), struggled to structure, categorize, and even recall how they made the moment-to-moment decisions that inform their actions.

On reflection, mindful of the experiences shared by readers, we realized more structure was needed to make completing the exercise possible. In consultations, we found ourselves suggesting a framework presented by Marvin Goldfried (1980) in his classic article, "Toward the Delineation of Therapeutic Change Principles." There, he recommended conceptualizing one's therapeutic work as "involving various levels of abstraction":

> At the highest level . . . we have the *theoretical framework* to explain how and why change takes place, as well as an accompanying *philosophical stance* on the nature of human functioning. . . . At the lowest level . . ., we have therapeutic *techniques* or clinical *procedures* that are actually employed during the intervention process. . . . [To these, add] a level of abstraction somewhere between theory and technique which, for want of a better term, we might call *clinical strategies* . . . [or] *principles* of change . . . clinical heuristics that implicitly guide our efforts during the course of therapy. (p. 994, italics in original)

Goldfried's (1980) three levels of abstraction are listed from highest to lowest in Table 1.1, which can serve as a template for creating a blueprint of your therapeutic approach. To these, a fourth can be added. Termed "metatheory," it is a higher order concept representing the assumptions on which our theories are based. With regard to psychotherapy, Wampold (2001) identified two. The first, commonly known as the medical model, posits the efficacy of psychotherapy depends on the clinical procedure being specifically remedial to the

TABLE 1.1. Goldfried's Levels of Abstraction

Level of abstraction	How is this represented in your work?		
	Beginning	Middle	End
Metatheory			
Theoretical framework			
Clinical strategies			
Techniques			

Note. Data from Goldfried (1980).

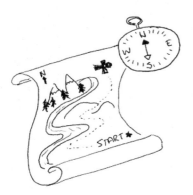

FIELD GUIDE TIP

Need help with a concrete example of applying Goldfried's classification to a popular therapeutic approach? Turn to pages 54–56 in Chapter 3.

disorder being treated. The second, the contextual model, holds the benefits of psychotherapy primarily accrue through social processes characteristic of all human interaction (e.g., relationship, connection, shared beliefs and values, negotiated agreements, persuasion).

If you have not already done so, take the time now to create your therapy blueprint using the framework provided. Recreating the table in a spreadsheet makes the process easy and ensures ample space for details and future modifications. As you do so, note how the various levels come into play at different points—beginning, middle, and end—in your performance of psychotherapy.

Getting to the Source of Your Success (Part 2)

With your blueprint in hand, the next step is to identify how your work—from start to finish and across the levels of abstraction—leverages the five factors responsible for outcome (i.e., client and extratherapeutic factors, alliance and relationship, therapist effects, hope and expectancy, and structure). Make a note if and when you find presuppositions, beliefs, or actions that may impede, obstruct, or undermine or cannot be directly connected to any of the factors (see Table 1.2). Completing this exercise now will help you use the TDPA to identify those DP activities with the greatest potential for improving your effectiveness.

Recall, as discussed in *BR*, time and experience lead to the development of automaticity (pp. 27–29). We literally become able to act without thinking. While enhancing efficiency, the problem, Ericsson (2006a) pointed out, is we "lose conscious control over the production of [our] actions" (p. 694). We literally do not remember *how* we do what we do. As a result, our ability to make specific intentional adjustments to our work is compromised.

Regaining consciousness is a necessary first step—one, experience shows, many find challenging. If you are struggling to complete your blueprint or connect your work to the five factors, consider starting with a smaller task, such as

- *reviewing a recent treatment plan and clinical notes;*
- *recording and reviewing a session, taking time to note your decisions and actions; and*
- *reflecting on a conversation with a colleague in which you discussed a case, noting the words you used and what you emphasized and omitted from your description.*

TABLE 1.2. Connecting Your Work to the Factors With the Right Stuff

Level of abstraction	How is this represented in your work, and what factor is being leveraged?		
	Beginning	Middle	End
Metatheory			
Theoretical framework			
Clinical strategies			
Techniques			

Principle 4: Keep Your Eyes on the Next Step

Appreciating Each Step

The evidence is clear. Nearly 90% of clinicians are "highly motivated" to transcend their current level of performance. The problem is improving effectiveness comes slowly, with the pace of progress dramatically disproportionate to the time and effort required. To combat the risk of giving up, learn to prize each accomplishment along the way. Toward this end, reflect on an earlier accomplishment (e.g., playing a musical instrument, learning a new language, finishing college or graduate school):

- *Create a timeline of the decisions, choices, and actions leading up to your achievement.*
- *In as much detail as possible, recall how you felt as you reached each milestone.*
- *Note how you addressed setbacks or failures you encountered before reaching your objective.*
- *What role did others play (or not) in addressing setbacks or failures encountered while reaching for your objective?*
- *Describe how you thought about your final objective at each step along the way.*

Now, take a moment to reflect on a time when you started out but stopped before reaching your final objective (e.g., playing a musical instrument, learning a new language or skill, writing an article or book):

- *Create a timeline of the decisions, choices, and actions leading up to when you stopped.*
- *In as much detail as possible, recall how you felt as you reached each milestone.*
- *Note how you addressed setbacks or failures you encountered before reaching your objective.*
- *Describe how you thought about your final objective at each step along the way.*
- *List any differences between the time you stopped and when you reached your objective in how you approached each step.*

Word Work

DP is inherently incremental and cumulative. Progress comes in a series of small steps instead of a sudden, dramatic, or radical change in how you work. As such, preparation, pacing, patience, and endurance are key. Bearing this in mind, take a moment to imagine you are planning to participate in a marathon:

- *List as many words that come to mind about what you need to prepare to complete the race.*

Now, imagine you will be participating in a sprint (e.g., 50 or 100 meters):

- *List as many words that come to mind about what you need to prepare for to maximize your performance.*

1. Note the differences between the words you generated, striking any the two lists have in common. With your plan to apply DP to your professional development in mind, develop one strategy for each unique word you associated with preparing for a marathon.

DECISION POINT

What to do next:

- If you have sufficient performance data for analysis but have yet to use the TDPA to develop a specific, individualized learning objective, turn to Chapter 2.

- If you have used the TDPA to establish a specific, individualized learning objective but are struggling to stay focused or motivated, turn to Chapter 8.

- If you have completed the TDPA and need help developing a DP exercise for your specific objective, turn to
  - Chapter 3 for client factors
  - Chapter 4 for therapist factors
  - Chapter 5 for relationship factors
  - Chapter 6 for hope and expectancy factors
  - Chapter 7 for structure

REFERENCES

Adams, S. (2013). *How to fail at almost everything and still win big: Kind of the story of my life*. Penguin Random House.

American Psychological Association. (2017). *Ethical principles of psychologists and code of conduct* (2002, amended effective June 1, 2010, and January 1, 2017). https://www.apa.org/ethics/code/index.aspx

Amirault, R. J., & Branson, K. R. (2006). Educators and expertise: A brief history of theories and models. In K. A. Ericsson, N. Charness, P. J. Feltovich, & R. R. Hoffman (Eds.), *The Cambridge handbook of expertise and expert performance* (pp. 69–86). Cambridge University Press.

Barnes, A. (1981). *Barnes notes on the old and new testaments: An explanatory and practical commentary*. Baker Book House.

Bike, D. H., Norcross, J. C., & Schatz, D. M. (2009). Processes and outcomes of psychotherapists' personal therapy: Replication and extension 20 years later. *Psychotherapy, 46*(1), 19–31. https://doi.org/10.1037/a0015139

Brattland, H., Koksvik, J. M., Burkeland, O., Gråwe, R. W., Klöckner, C., Linaker, O. M., Ryum, T., Wampold, B., Lara-Cabrera, M. L., & Iversen, V. C. (2018). The effects of routine outcome monitoring (ROM) on therapy outcomes in the course of an implementation process: A randomized clinical trial. *Journal of Counseling Psychology, 65*(5), 641–652. https://doi.org/10.1037/cou0000286

Bunzeck, N., & Düzel, E. (2006). Absolute coding of stimulus novelty in the human substantia nigra/VTA. *Neuron, 51*(3), 369–379. https://doi.org/10.1016/j.neuron.2006.06.021

Caldwell, B. E. (2015). *Saving psychotherapy: How therapists can bring the talking cure back from the brink*. Benjamin Caldwell.

Chow, D., & Miller, S. D. (2022). *Taxonomy of Deliberate Practice Activities in Psychotherapy—Therapist Version* (Version 6). International Center for Clinical Excellence.

Chow, D. L., Miller, S. D., Seidel, J. A., Kane, R. T., Thornton, J. A., & Andrews, W. P. (2015). The role of deliberate practice in the development of highly effective psychotherapists. *Psychotherapy, 52*(3), 337–345. https://doi.org/10.1037/pst0000015

Chow, L., Miller, K., & Jones, H. (2022). *Improving difficult conversations in therapy: A randomized trial of a deliberate practice training program* [Manuscript submitted for publication]. International Center for Clinical Excellence, Chicago, IL.

Colvin, G. (2008). *Talent is overrated: What really separates world-class performers from everybody else.* Nicholas Brealey.

de Jong, K., van Sluis, P., Nugter, M. A., Heiser, W. J., & Spinhoven, P. (2012). Understanding the differential impact of outcome monitoring: Therapist variables that moderate feedback effects in a randomized clinical trial. *Psychotherapy Research, 22*(4), 464–474. https://doi.org/10.1080/10503307.2012.673023

Ericsson, A., & Pool, R. (2016). *Peak: Secrets from the new science of expertise.* Houghton Mifflin Harcourt.

Ericsson, K. A. (2006a). The influence of experience and deliberate practice on the development of superior performance. In K. A. Ericsson, N. Charness, P. Feltovich, & R. Hoffman (Eds.), *The Cambridge handbook of expertise and expert performance* (pp. 683–701). Cambridge University Press.

Ericsson, K. A. (2006b). An introduction to the Cambridge handbook of expertise and expert performance: Its development, organization, and content. In K. A. Ericsson, N. Charness, P. J. Feltovich, & R. R. Hoffman (Eds.), *The Cambridge handbook of expertise and expert performance* (pp. 3–20). Cambridge University Press. https://doi.org/10.1017/CBO9780511816796.001

Ericsson, K. A., Krampe, R. T., & Tesch-Romer, C. (1993). The role of deliberate practice in the acquisition of expert performance. *Psychological Review, 100*(3), 363–406. https://doi.org/10.1037/0033-295X.100.3.363

Germer, S., Weyrich, V., Bräscher, A.-K., Mütze, K., & Witthöft, M. (2022). Does practice really make perfect? A longitudinal analysis of the relationship between therapist experience and therapy outcome: A replication of Goldberg, Rousmaniere, et al. (2016). *Journal of Counseling Psychology, 69*(5), 745–754. https://doi.org/10.1037/cou0000608

Goldberg, S. B., Rousmaniere, T., Miller, S. D., Whipple, J., Nielsen, S. L., Hoyt, W. T., & Wampold, B. E. (2016). Do psychotherapists improve with time and experience? A longitudinal analysis of outcomes in a clinical setting. *Journal of Counseling Psychology, 63*(1), 1–11. https://doi.org/10.1037/cou0000131

Goldfried, M. R. (1980). Toward the delineation of therapeutic change principles. *American Psychologist, 35*(11), 991–999. https://doi.org/10.1037/0003-066X.35.11.991

Hatfield, D. R., & Ogles, B. M. (2007). Why some clinicians use outcome measures and others do not. *Administration and Policy in Mental Health, 34*(3), 283–291. https://doi.org/10.1007/s10488-006-0110-y

Hubble, M. A., Duncan, B. L., & Miller, S. D. (1999). Introduction. In M. A. Hubble, B. L. Duncan, & S. D. Miller (Eds.), *The heart and soul of change: What works in therapy* (pp. 1–19). American Psychological Association.

Info Learners. (2022, April 9). *How hard is it to get into grad school for psychology.* https://infolearners.com/how-hard-is-it-to-get-into-grad-school-for-psychology/

Karamanou, M., Panayiotakopoulos, G., Tsoucalas, G., Kousoulis, A. A., & Androutsos, G. (2012). From miasmas to germs: A historical approach to theories of infectious disease transmission. *Le Infezioni in Medicina, 20*(1), 58–62.

Madsen, J., Markova, V., Hernandez, L., Tomfohr-Madsen, L. M., & Miller, S. D. (2021). Training practices in routine outcome monitoring among accredited psychology doctoral programs in Canada. *Training and Education in Professional Psychology.* Advance online publication. https://doi.org/10.1037/tep0000389

Mathewes, B., & Miller, S. D. (2020, January/February). Meet me at McGinnis Meadows. *Psychotherapy Networker, 44,* 46–57.

Miller, S. D., Hubble, M. A., & Chow, D. (2020). *Better results: Using deliberate practice to improve therapeutic effectiveness.* American Psychological Association. https://doi.org/10.1037/0000191-000

Miller, S. D., Hubble, M. A., Chow, D., & Seidel, J. (2015). Beyond measures and monitoring: Realizing the potential of feedback-informed treatment. *Psychotherapy*, *52*(4), 449–457. https://doi.org/10.1037/pst0000031

Miller, S. D., Hubble, M. A., & Duncan, B. L. (2007). Supershrinks: What's the secret of their success? *Psychotherapy Networker*, *31*(6).

Miller, S. D., Madsen, J., & Hubble, M. A. (2020). Toward an evidence-based standard of professional competence. In M. Trachsel, J. Gaab, N. Biller-Andorno, S. Tekin, & J. Sadler (Eds.), *Oxford handbook of psychotherapy ethics* (pp. 951–968). Oxford University Press.

Minami, T., Wampold, B. E., Serlin, R. C., Hamilton, E. G., Brown, G. S., & Kircher, J. C. (2008). Benchmarking the effectiveness of psychotherapy treatment for adult depression in a managed care environment: A preliminary study. *Journal of Consulting and Clinical Psychology*, *76*(1), 116–124. https://doi.org/10.1037/0022-006X.76.1.116

Neimeyer, G. J., & Taylor, J. M. (2011). Continuing education in psychology. In J. C. Norcross, G. R. VandenBos, & D. K. Freedheim (Eds.), *History of psychotherapy: Continuity and change* (2nd ed., pp. 663–672). American Psychological Association. https://doi.org/10.1037/12353-043

Neimeyer, G. J., Taylor, J. M., & Wear, D. M. (2009). Continuing education in psychology: Outcomes, evaluations, and mandates. *Professional Psychology, Research and Practice*, *40*(6), 617–624. https://doi.org/10.1037/a0016655

Nissen-Lie, H. A., Monsen, J. T., & Rønnestad, M. H. (2010). Therapist predictors of early patient-rated working alliance: A multilevel approach. *Psychotherapy Research*, *20*(6), 627–646. https://doi.org/10.1080/10503307.2010.497633

Nissen-Lie, H. A., & Rønnestad, M. H. (2016). The empirical evidence for psychotherapist humility as a foundation for psychotherapist expertise. *Psychotherapy Bulletin*, *51*, 7–9.

Norcross, J. C. (2005). The psychotherapist's own psychotherapy: Educating and developing psychologists. *American Psychologist*, *60*(8), 840–850. https://doi.org/10.1037/0003-066X.60.8.840

Orlinsky, D. E., & Rønnestad, M. H. (2005). *How psychotherapists develop: A study of therapeutic work and professional growth.* American Psychological Association. https://doi.org/10.1037/11157-000

Prochaska, J. O., Norcross, J. C., & Saul, S. F. (2020). Generating psychotherapy breakthroughs: Transtheoretical strategies from population health psychology. *American Psychologist*, *75*(7), 996–1010. https://doi.org/10.1037/amp0000568

Reese, R. J., Duncan, B. L., Bohanske, R. T., Owen, J. J., & Minami, T. (2014). Benchmarking outcomes in a public behavioral health setting: Feedback as a quality improvement strategy. *Journal of Consulting and Clinical Psychology*, *82*(4), 731–742. https://doi.org/10.1037/a0036915

Saxon, D., & Barkham, M. (2012). Patterns of therapist variability: Therapist effects and the contribution of patient severity and risk. *Journal of Consulting and Clinical Psychology*, *80*(4), 535–546. Advance online publication. https://doi.org/10.1037/a0028898

Stiles, W. B., Barkham, M., Mellor-Clark, J., & Connell, J. (2008). Effectiveness of cognitive-behavioural, person-centred, and psychodynamic therapies in UK primary-care routine practice: Replication in a larger sample. *Psychological Medicine*, *38*(5), 677–688. https://doi.org/10.1017/S0033291707001511

Tao, K. W., Owen, J., Pace, B. T., & Imel, Z. E. (2015). A meta-analysis of multicultural competencies and psychotherapy process and outcome. *Journal of Counseling Psychology*, *62*(3), 337–350. https://doi.org/10.1037/cou0000086

Wampold, B. E. (2001). *The great psychotherapy debate: Models, methods, and findings.* Erlbaum.

Wampold, B. E., & Imel, Z. E. (2015). *The great psychotherapy debate: The evidence for what makes psychotherapy work* (2nd ed.). Routledge/Taylor & Francis Group.

2

Identifying and Refining Your Individualized Learning Objective

Daryl Chow, Scott D. Miller, and Mark A. Hubble

Truth, like gold, is to be obtained not by its growth, but by washing away from it all that is not gold.

—LEO TOLSTOY, *TOLSTOY'S DIARIES*

DECISION POINT

Begin here if you have read the book *Better Results* and

- are routinely measuring your performance *and*

- have collected sufficient data to establish a reliable, evidence-based profile of your therapeutic effectiveness *or*

- have created a map or blueprint of how you work sufficiently detailed another clinician could step into your shoes *and*

- need guidance using the Taxonomy of Deliberate Practice Activities in Psychotherapy to identify or refine an individualized learning objective with the greatest chance of improving your effectiveness.

https://doi.org/10.1037/0000358-003
The Field Guide to Better Results: Evidence-Based Exercises to Improve Therapeutic Effectiveness,
S. D. Miller, D. Chow, S. Malins, and M. A. Hubble (Editors)

o begin, please rate your response to each of the following questions on a scale from 1 to 5, where 1 is *highly disagree* and 5 *highly agree*:

- You are someone who is often attuned to the feelings of others.

- You are someone who approaches life, work, and problems systematically and sequentially, often having clearly defined steps and procedures in mind (i.e., "If x, then y").

Not surprisingly, psychotherapists tend to assign a 4 or 5 to the first statement and lower scores to the second. Clearly, possessing an empathic disposition helps in fulfilling the desire to be of assistance to people in distress. Being in the moment, emphasizing understanding and acceptance, placing trust in feelings, and relying on intuition to guide decision making are often given priority in the daily conduct of therapy. Carefully constructing a treatment plan, following an established protocol, and being able to state clearly and explicitly the rationale for each and every action taken with clients is less common. On balance, therapists are more *empathizers* than *systemizers*.

As it is, being completely immersed in and sharply attuned to the client's experience has long been regarded as the sine qua non of expert clinical work. Indeed, a large multinational investigation by the University of Chicago's David Orlinsky and the University of Oslo's Michael Rønnestad (2005), involving more than 10,000 therapists, found the majority not only yearn for but also consider the experience of connecting deeply with clients the quintessence of what it means to be a therapist. For all that, *healing involvement*—the term used by researchers to characterize this belief and desire—has a curious relationship with results. The more it is valued, the *less* effective one is likely to be. In reality, the best clinicians rate it significantly less important to their work and identity than their more average counterparts (Chow, 2014). What holds their attention and gets them up and going in the morning? Outcome.

Enter the Taxonomy of Deliberate Practice Activities in Psychotherapy (TDPA; Chow & Miller, 2022; see Appendix A, this volume), the tool specifically designed to help practitioners develop a step-by-step professional development plan most likely to improve their results. Unfortunately, a cursory review of the document is likely to strike empathizers as, in a word, foreign. A spreadsheet of tables, ratings, and detailed instructions has replaced what they do best, know the most about, and hold in the highest esteem: connection, caring, intuition, and being in the moment. How can the seemingly detached, calculating, even antiseptic nature of the TDPA be experienced as anything other than off-putting?

Turns out, the answer—and the way forward—lies in redefining what healing involvement encompasses. Nowhere is the need to do so more apparent than in efforts to address the epidemic levels of burnout seen in the helping professions. The terms *vicarious trauma, secondary traumatic stress,* and especially *compassion fatigue* all point to the very real risks of deriving meaning and purpose primarily from the emotionally charged interactions during the therapy hour— especially with nonimproving clients. The pattern is as easy to see as the results are predictable: In the face of continued suffering, deepening involvement feels like the right thing to do.

And yet, as Mathieu and colleagues (2015) pointed out, "Burnout doesn't begin with caring, or even caring too much, but continuing to care *ineffectively* [emphasis added], losing sight of what we're there to accomplish with our clients in the first place" (p. 22). Little wonder the panoply of recommendations offered by burnout experts—including cultivating mindfulness, going on walks, doing yoga, joining a service organization, turning off technology, capping client contact hours, and eliminating caffeine and alcohol intake—do not work. All miss that key protective factor—doing something that *actually helps*. Recall feeling effective is so crucial to the well-being of therapists, they routinely over-estimate their actual results (see Chow et al., 2015; Lin et al., 2022; Walfish et al., 2012)!

Thus, it is essential for the definition of healing involvement to be extended beyond the immediate experience with the client to therapists' deeply felt desire to be of help. With this perspective in mind, "empathizers" can transform the TDPA from a mere chore to a deep and powerful act of caring. At this stage, it is recommended therapists work consciously and intentionally at developing a relationship, with achieving better results equal to the relationships one works so hard to establish and maintain with clients.

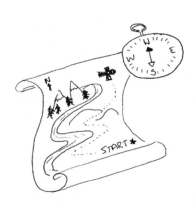

FIELD GUIDE TIP

Readers who scored a 4 or 5 on the second statement (i.e., systemizer) or who, after reading *Better Results* (Miller et al., 2020), are now looking for tips, suggestions, and practical guidance for maximizing the utility of the TDPA may feel free to skip ahead to the exercises at the end of this chapter.

BARRIERS TO BETTER RESULTS

To be clear, it is not that therapists do *not* want to improve. They do. The evidence reviewed in Chapter 12 of *Better Results* (*BR*; Miller et al., 2020) proves it. However, for empathizers and systemizers alike, three obstacles get in the way of deepening their relationship with better results:

- what therapists already believe works,
- not knowing what will work to improve their effectiveness, and
- what others insist works if only everyone would do it.

Regarding the last item on the list, nothing beyond the decades of research reviewed in Chapter 2 of *BR* and the first chapter of this volume need be repeated. The desire to help those in psychological pain is easily exploited by those promising a better way. In the busy, time-and-resource-limited world in which clinicians work, one of the major hooks is, "The heavy lifting has been done. All you need to do is follow directions." If this remains a temptation, complete the exercises on page 17 of Chapter 1 under Principle 1 (Avoid the Athenian Trap).

Turning to the first item, the evidence paints a rather bleak picture. Despite participating in continuing education throughout one's career, clinician confidence increases but their outcomes do not (Germer et al., 2022; Goldberg et al., 2016). Effective deliberate practice (DP) is predicated on developing an evidence-based profile of each therapist's effectiveness. The goal is to strengthen what one does well and target particular weaknesses for improvement. In either case, the expertise literature definitively shows intuition is not a reliable guide (Miller et al., 2018).

Finally, not knowing what to work on is a major obstacle—perhaps the biggest. It is also the reason for and purpose of this chapter. Consider the data presented in Figure 2.1. Displayed are the responses of hundreds of participants from an ongoing series of asynchronous, web-based trainings on DP conducted by the authors since the publication of *BR*. Asked at the outset of the course to identify the single biggest challenge attendees faced in their professional development, the majority (~38%) cited not knowing which goals or performance objectives to pursue.

The promise of the TDPA (as originally introduced in *BR*) was that completing the tool would help each therapist identify the specific DP activity exerting the greatest leverage on improving their results (McChesney et al., 2012). Experience showed clinicians needed more. Putting all the pieces together and arriving at a single professional development objective proved to be a

FIGURE 2.1. Responses From Deliberate Practice Web-Based Workshop

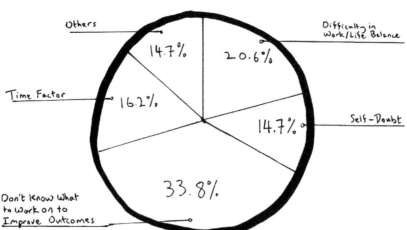

"bridge too far," at times eluding even the most dedicated. The sheer volume of information made it easy to get lost in the details, obscuring connections between the various inputs and, ultimately, the bigger picture.

KEEPING THE BIGGER PICTURE IN MIND

Step back for a moment. The journey is a series of steps for deepening involvement with better results, beginning with creating a detailed blueprint of how one works (see Figure 2.2). Recall the blueprint is a guide on "how you do, what you do" in therapy. A useful way to think about this is to imagine explaining to someone what you do within the therapy hour. As introduced in *BR* and thoroughly described in Chapter 1 of this field guide (*FG*), the reason for doing so is to enable the clinician to pinpoint where in their work they can intervene once they have identified what needs to change. The next step is measurement, routinely assessing engagement and outcome. The purpose is to generate data sufficient for the therapist to identify any weaknesses or deficits in their clinical performance. Once known, completing the TDPA is supposed to, first, help the therapist link their specific shortcomings to the factor or factors (and associated clinical activities) having the greatest chance of improving their results and, second, to develop a single, well-defined, and achievable professional development goal.

All well and good. Except . . .

Integrating data about one's performance deficits with the TDPA is where many end up feeling stuck. Consider the example of Liam.[1] First, he created a blueprint for his approach to clinical work. It took a while to fill in the details over time as he reflected on and conducted therapy. At the same time,

FIGURE 2.2. The Deliberate Practice Journey

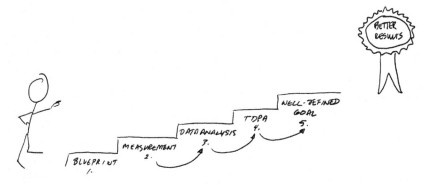

Note. TDPA = Taxonomy of Deliberate Practice Activities in Psychotherapy.

---

[1]All case examples used in the *FG* are composites of real people whose identifying information has been altered to ensure anonymity.

he began administering standardized measures to his clients. Once sufficient data were gathered for a reliable assessment of his work, he learned his impact—as reflected in his effect size—was average. Wanting to improve nonetheless, he turned to the TDPA. Instead of leading him to a specific target for DP, variable scores within each of the five factors (i.e., structure, hope and expectancy, relationship, client, therapist) left him puzzled about where to start. Frustrated, he turned to colleagues in his consultation group: "What am I supposed to do to get better?"

Experience shows Liam's struggle is far from unusual. Recall most therapists are average. As such, an *initial* examination of one's overall results often fails to reveal the one truly transformative DP objective. Instead of returning to the data with different and more detailed questions, many place their trust in the TDPA, hoping it will provide direction. Occasionally, when completed together with a coach, potential targets for improvement are identified. However, more often than not—as in the case of Liam—nothing specific stands out. In either instance, disconnected from performance data, both risk investing significant effort for an unknown return.

Recalling the advice offered earlier, the key to success is to treat the process of arriving at a performance improvement objective the same way one approaches working with clients. Get involved. Dive in, care, be curious, make connections, think critically, test understandings, continuously adapt, and, when required, seek consultation. No therapist thinks of "getting to know" the client as an activity independent of treatment. Similarly, learning what one needs to learn (and learn next) is not a precursor to but an integral part of DP. Practically speaking, this means returning to earlier steps as often as needed with different questions in mind:

- Is my blueprint accurate? Does it reliably capture how I work?

- Have I created an atmosphere that supports and facilitates candid feedback from clients? How do I use client feedback to inform and improve my work?

- How well do I understand my performance-related data? What gives rise to the numbers in the report? What variations in my performance (e.g., types of clients, presenting concerns, times of day, days of the week, treatment delivery format) might be hidden in the aggregate statistics?

- How does the information from my map, ongoing measurement, performance data, and the TDPA tie together? What am I learning about myself, how I work, with whom, and under what circumstances I am most and least effective?

Liam sought out a coach who encouraged him to set aside the TDPA temporarily and revisit his performance data. Specifically, as suggested in Chapter 10 of *BR*, he was encouraged to begin parsing his outcomes, linking them to a variety of factors known to be associated with variations in therapist effectiveness (i.e., level of client distress, amount of improvement over time, culture, gender or sexual orientation, quality of the alliance, and presenting problem).

To this end, Liam created a spreadsheet. On the vertical axis, he listed his clients and, horizontally, the various factors. It took him the better part of a month to pull the specific data points for each client and place them in the appropriate column and row. Importantly, as he did so, he had no preconceived ideas about what he might find. Once complete, however, a pattern immediately jumped out. His poorest outcomes occurred with men. "Was this the answer?" he wondered. "Should I get some training on 'men's' issues? Supervision?" Feeling uncertain, he returned to the coach.

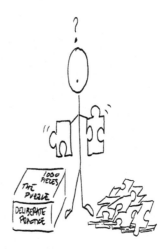

Together, they first examined the other dimensions in the spreadsheet, looking for connections and relationships. No other patterns stood out. The poor results weren't linked to the alliance, presenting problem, or differences in background or culture. Simply put, some men fared worse than others. "So, what is it I'm supposed to practice?" Liam asked, exasperated. The coach immediately replied, "Being curious. We're not done getting to know these men, what happens when you are with them, what it is about them." It was then the coach suggested Liam add a column to his spreadsheet. There, he was instructed to review his progress notes, tracking any recurring words used when documenting his work.

"I've figured it out!" Liam happily reported the following month: "I need to deliberately practice working with angry men—that's the word that showed up again and again in my notes: angry." Liam's experience highlights the need to modify the picture most people have of DP (see Figure 2.3). Rarely linear and sequential, more often than not, it is a matter of three steps forward and two back—and Liam had a couple more steps back ahead of him.

Retrieving the TDPA, the coach wondered how best to understand the anger reported in Liam's notes. Was a description of the men, their nature, and how they presented a client factor? Or was it a result of something taking place in the therapeutic interaction (i.e., relationship factor)? There is one more

FIGURE 2.3. Deliberate Practice: What People Think and What It Really Looks Like

SUCCESS

WHAT PEOPLE THINK IT LOOKS LIKE

SUCCESS

WHAT IT REALLY LOOKS LIKE

possibility: Was it a therapist factor? Did Liam somehow evoke an angry response from certain men? If so, what was it about him?

With these questions in mind, Liam returned to his notes. In short order, he discovered the problem was not "angry men." Rather, those with the poorest results *became* angry when they were not getting what they wanted: advice and direction, two activities conspicuously missing in Liam's blueprint.

"I'm not comfortable telling people what to do," he observed at the next session with his coach, adding, "In fact, I was trained *not* to do that." At this point, and after months of work, a DP objective likely to have leverage on Liam's outcomes started to emerge. Along the way, several shifts in perspective had occurred. What began abstractly as "men's issues" (TDPA Dimension 4) turned into "relating to angry men" (Dimension 3, Di, ii) but eventually landed on the necessity of being aware of and accommodating the expectations of certain men (Dimension 4b, c). With the correct focus sorted, Liam was finally able to act, devoting attention to learning when, with whom, and under what circumstances being more direct and offering specific guidance were indicated. In time, he modified his therapeutic map to reflect his new understandings.

PRINCIPLES FOR IDENTIFYING AND REFINING YOUR INDIVIDUALIZED LEARNING OBJECTIVE

Three principles essential to developing a learning objective with the greatest chance of improving your effectiveness are suggested. Derived from experiences working with clinicians like Liam since the publication of *BR*, they include

- approaching finding your performance improvement objective with the same interest and dedication you devote to understanding your clients,
- treating the process of arriving at your performance improvement objective as an ongoing learning project, and
- focusing on the "what," and the "know-how" will follow.

Up to this point, the aim of the entire chapter has been operationalizing the first two principles—what identifying your specific performance objective *actually* entails and the perspective required to sustain your efforts along the way. What more can be said? Like getting to know your clients, no shortcuts exist. Hopefully, it is clear DP is not an event (or even a series of discrete events). It is an ongoing, *iterative* process. Arrival is not possible without the journey—and in the case of working to achieve better results, it is best to think of the two as one and the same. You are here now. What are you learning? What is next?

Whereas the first two principles direct attention to the importance of attitude, Principle 3 is less about one's point of view than how the task is best approached. Toward this end, a specific framework for conceptualizing and organizing your efforts to identify the "what" and "how" to DP has proven useful. Known by the acronym OPL, it contains three elements: outcome goal, process goal, and learning project (see Figure 2.4).

Of the three, the learning project has already been introduced and illustrated with an example. Its purpose is to fill in gaps in knowledge. Its nature is dynamic, flexible, and exploratory. That said, effective learning projects share three qualities. First, the environment is conducive to learning and relearning, retrieving and reflecting on prior knowledge, and ultimately transferring what is being learned into clinical practice (Ahrens, 2017; Chow, 2019a; Haskell, 2001). As recommended in *BR*, one important strategy is actively working to protect the time one sets aside for DP (e.g., turning off the phone, social media, and email notifications, including other interruptions). Second, effective learning projects are open to a wide variety of inputs. That means looking beyond the world of therapy for inspiration and guidance. For example, if creating more effective structure in sessions is the objective, "know-how" might come from a colleague or therapy book but also from watching a documentary on how filmmakers craft the narrative arch of a story to create emotional impact. Third, and last, mindful of "Parkinson's Law"— the danger that when left open-ended, work will expand to fill the time allotted—the most productive learning projects are time bound. As simplistic as it may seem, Liam was given specific tasks to complete within a given period, allowing him and his coach to monitor progress easily, make needed "just-in-time" adjustments, and plan the next steps.

It goes without saying that learning projects are goal directed. Goals both inform and determine the learning project. Returning to Figure 2.4, the first, or outcome goal, is "what" one aims to achieve in the learning project. Recall that Liam's initial objective was to improve his results. When his attention shifted to the "how," or process goal, the initial outcome goal evolved—first, from improving results with men to becoming eventually more comfortable and skilled in working with men who wanted and expected direction and advice. Once clear, the items listed in the TDPA provide numerous evidence-based suggestions for effective action. As portrayed in the graphic, think of the process goal as a lever. Its purpose is to provide the structure (i.e., lift) to reach the desired outcome.

FIGURE 2.4. The OPL Framework

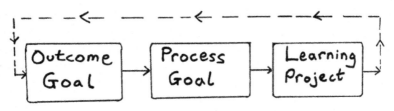

PRINCIPLE-BASED EXERCISES

Before considering the following exercises, ensure you have taken all the steps outlined in the decision tree presented at the start of this chapter. It is assumed you (a) are routinely measuring your performance; (b) have collected sufficient data to establish a reliable, evidence-based profile of your therapeutic effectiveness; (c) have created a map or blueprint sufficiently detailed so that another clinician could replicate your work; and (d) have tried to complete the TDPA but want additional help to develop the learning objective with the greatest chance of improving your effectiveness.

Have your outcome data, blueprint, and TDPA in front of you while determining which ones will work best for you. If, after considering the suggested exercises, you still find yourself struggling with outcome goals, process goals, and a learning project, consult the suggestions and detailed case example at the end of the chapter.

Exercise 1: Connecting With Your Authentic Self

Principle: 1
Applicability: TDPA Items 3Aiv, 3Biv, 5Avi
Purpose

People routinely equate authenticity with acting in a manner consistent with their *actual* selves. For all that, research indicates the experience most often arises when we think and act in ways consistent with our *ideal* self (Gan & Chen, 2017). As already stated, for many psychotherapists—especially those who principally see themselves as empathizers—data, statistics, and performance metrics evoke strong feelings of "not me." This exercise is designed to honor and reconnect you with the ideals that brought you to the field—being of service to others.

Task

Part 1. Set aside 20 minutes once or twice a week for 1 month to think about a person you hold in high esteem because of who they are and what they do. It could be anyone from any domain of human performance—an athlete, scientist, musician, philanthropist, a person from the present, or perhaps a historical figure. "Spend time with them" by looking up their accomplishments, listening to interviews, watching videos online, reading a biography, or imagining a conversation with them. Complete this part of the exercise before reading further.

Part 2. After a month, devote the same amount of time over several weeks to imagining how others would know that data-driven DP is part of your ideal self. Using paper and pencil or your favorite note-keeping app, maintain a record of your thoughts and reflections. Be as specific as possible about what you would be doing; how others would know your work with statistics, metrics, and data is critical to being the most helpful you can be. Last, make engaging in this exercise routine.

Exercise 2: Recovering Your "University Days" Mindset

Principle: 2
Applicability: Potentially All Items on the TDPA
Purpose

Going to college is more than earning a degree and getting a job. It's about exploration, self-discovery, learning to tolerate boredom, being exposed to diverse peoples and ideas, making friends, falling in love, and having fun. It is noteworthy that most who start end up studying a subject entirely different from what they originally planned—around 80%, actually (The University of Tulsa, 2020). Such shifts in interest and focus are both difficult to anticipate and far from an indication of failure, given their dependence on chance and experience. Of course, graduation is the ultimate objective (i.e., outcome goal). And yet, relishing the journey—its fits and starts, ups and downs, twists and turns—makes earning a degree rewarding and transformational. The same may be said of DP.

Task

Part 1. Set aside 20 minutes once or twice a week for 1 month to think about a person, class, relationship, book, time of life, or event that unexpectedly but positively impacted the direction of your career and life. Keep a log of your reflections, noting the circumstances, any challenges arising from the change in direction, and what was required of you to step off your then-current path and make it so (see Exercise 7). Consider how the change both confirmed or disrupted your sense of self up to that time.

Part 2. When it comes to your DP learning project, suspend the desire for an immediate result (i.e., being given a degree before the education). Cultivate a "university mindset." For the following month, be open to chance change-producing events, people, and experiences related to your desire to improve your therapeutic effectiveness. Keep a log using index cards or a note-keeping app. Return to this exercise whenever you embark on a new learning project.

Exercise 3: Specifying the Outcome Goal

Principle: 2, 3
Applicability: Potentially All Items on the TDPA
Purpose

The purpose of DP is different from attempting to resolve a difficult or "stuck" case. The latter is typically focused on anomalies or outliers, one-off experiences from which little can be learned or applied to other clients and contexts (in *BR*, referred to as random errors). The former is about identifying and addressing recurring patterns in one's behavior that consistently undermine effective performance (i.e., nonrandom errors). Doing so requires gathering data via routine outcome monitoring sufficient to offer a reliable and valid profile of one's strengths and weaknesses. Once done, patterns can be extracted and effectively targeted for performance improvement.

Task

Part 1. Solve for patterns. After you have collected outcome and relationship data on 40 to 60 cases:

1. Using "closed" cases only, partition your outcome data into "successful" versus "unsuccessful" groups.

2. Study the two groups, looking for differences (gender, age, presenting problem, strength of the relationship, amount and trajectory of change, consistencies in your thinking and feeling about the clients).

3. Spend no more than 20 minutes at any one sitting, allowing time in between for the information to "percolate." Jot down any observations, thoughts, or "aha's" that occur to you during the time away.

Part 2. The next step is separating committed from aspirational outcome goals. To do so,

1. List all potential targets for DP (i.e., outcome goals) based on the analysis completed in Part 1.

2. Compare your results with the performance benchmarks (*BR*, pages 74–75).

3. Get as specific as possible. For example,
   – Reduce my youth population dropout rates from 47% to below 20%.
   – Reduce deterioration rates for men from 12% to 6%.
   – Reduce the rates of clients who make an unplanned termination after the first session from 35% to 20%.
   – Improve the rate of reliable change improvement for clients who have not experienced improvement after being seen for more than six sessions from 50% to 60%.

4. Commit to one outcome goal, temporarily designating all others aspirational (Doerr, 2018). The one committed outcome goal is the single target to which you will devote your efforts. (The next exercises will help identify and refine the process goal and learning project.) A good rule to follow is picking "low hanging fruit"—something that has high leverage on improving your overall effectiveness while also being easy to reach.

Exercise 4: Figuring out Your Process Goal

Principle: 2, 3
Applicability: Potentially All Items on the TDPA
Purpose
Once you know your "what," the TDPA is specifically designed to help you figure out the "how" (i.e., your process goal). On the basis of feedback from therapists since the publication of *BR* and the research reviewed in the *FG*, significant revisions have been made to the tool.

Task

With your outcome goal in mind, review the latest version of the TDPA, taking time to

1. Rate each item. Spending time reviewing case notes from active clients will ensure accuracy and representativeness.

2. Go through the document and identify the top three activities you believe will have the greatest impact on your results.

3. Select one to work on now, making sure it is *influenceable* and *predictive* of the outcome goal you've listed (see Figure 2.5).

4. Have a coach or expert—someone who knows your work—complete the Supervisor/Coach version of the TDPA and compare the ratings. Work together to identify and design a single process goal.

Exercise 5: Antigoals

Principle: 2
Applicability: Potentially All Items on the TDPA
Purpose

Being clear about what is unimportant in our efforts to improve can be a powerful way to achieve clarity and maintain focus on our process goal.

Task

This exercise is simple yet effective. Review your completed TDPA, making a list of the items (and factors) that will *not* be a part of your primary process goal. Keep the list handy, reviewing it whenever you are tempted to pursue training or activities (outside of playful experimentations and just having fun) unrelated or tangential to your current process goal.

FIGURE 2.5. Influencing Outcome With a Process That Is Predictive and Influenceable

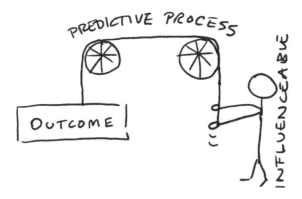

Exercise 6: Create a Centralized Note-Taking System

Principle: 1, 2, 3
Applicability: Potentially All Items on the TDPA
Purpose

Journaling and note taking, research indicates, has multiple benefits. A study in the *Journal of Experimental Psychology*, for example, found it reduced intrusive and avoidant thoughts about negative events while improving working memory (Klein & Boals, 2001). Such improvements, it is believed, free up precious (and limited) cognitive resources to focus on other mental activities (e.g., managing stress, maintaining focus, learning). While popular in the treatment and self-help literature, the benefits for anyone engaging in DP could not be clearer. Keeping a consistent and "centralized" (i.e., one fixed note-taking location) record helps in the recollection, organization, and consolidation of new learnings (Agarwal & Bain, 2019; Chow, 2019a; Miller et al., 2020). On the flip side, the lack of a centralized note-taking system is often a barrier to accelerated learning.

Task

Part 1. Determine how you will keep a record of your DP efforts (e.g., handwritten, using a note-taking app). In this record, document your experiences, including those that might strike you as irrelevant to your current learning project. Treat your record as a garden you must seed, nurture, nourish, and prune on an ongoing basis to bear fruit.

Here are some tips that others have found helpful:

- If you decide to keep handwritten notes:
  - Put them in a bound journal.
  - Number and date both the notebook and pages because doing so will help in recall.
  - Leave the first few pages blank to facilitate the later creation of a *map of content*. Unlike a traditional table of contents, the map of content is designed to both highlight where specific content can be found (e.g., "Learning Project 1 on improving structure in therapy; see pages, 4, 32, and 33") and also facilitate making connections between sections within and between notebooks.
  - Use sticky "flag tabs" to highlight themes (e.g., green for key learnings, yellow for points requiring further consideration, blue for interesting but less useful ideas and insights).

- If you choose to use an electronic medium:
  - It should be easy to use. Bells and whistles are less important than accessibility and simplicity.
  - It should be easy to search, retrieve, and, most important, create links between notes. Certain apps (e.g., Notion, Roam Research, Obsidian)

allow for linking one note to another as well as using links to reference and connect themes within the notes (i.e., bidirectional. For instructions on the use of Obsidian to link your notes, see https://darylchow.com/frontiers/rightforyou/).

 – Use tags, labeling each note to create relationships amid the content (e.g., #empathy, #dropout, #couplestherapy). Of course, storing the notes in themed folders can also help to organize content.

• For the purposes of your learning project, consider keeping a record of the following:

 – Each week, recall the people you worked with, recording one mistake and one success. Limit each entry to 140 characters to ensure consistency and efficiency (see https://darylchow.com/frontiers/weeklytherapylearnings/ for an example).

 – Note thoughts, reflections, and summaries of readings, movies, books, and podcasts you have encountered, whether or not they seem relevant to your current learning project.

 – Record client feedback. Although you likely record this in your case notes, keeping a record in a central location will help in making connections between the various sources of information related to your learning project.

Part 2. After creating and starting a note-taking system, the next step is engaging in what experts in the learning sciences call *retrieval practice* (Agarwal & Bain, 2019). In practical terms, this means revisiting your notes on a routine basis, first looking at the heading or tags and trying to recall the specifics, and then refreshing your memory by reading the entire entry. Turns out that "testing yourself to learn" as opposed to "teaching to the test" is a powerful way of deepening your knowledge and understanding. Researchers believe it disrupts the false sense of fluency that can develop when details and nuance are forgotten in the learning process (Bjork, 2011). As you do so, resist early temptations to come to a conclusion, instead allowing the information to percolate in the hopes of making "higher order units, or 'chunks,' for conceiving, understanding, and organizing" (Miller et al., 2020, p. 27).

JANICE AND THE GIANT OUTCOME GOAL

As an example of applying the preceding exercises, consider Janice, a therapist with about 7 years of clinical experience who worked in both inpatient and outpatient mental health clinics. Once she had enough cases for a reliable, evidence-based analysis of her clinical performance, she took up Exercise 3 (i.e., specifying the outcome goal). In an effort to identify the outcome goal with the most leverage on improving her results, she created a spreadsheet listing each client's data (i.e., outcome and relationship scores) and other details. In a separate column, a distinction was drawn between those she treated successfully (reliable improvement) and unsuccessfully (lack of reliable change, deteriorated, or dropped out after the first session). Next, with the spreadsheet open on her computer, she started reviewing the progress notes of her closed cases, "sorting for patterns."

Four were immediately apparent. First, many of the clients Janice treated unsuccessfully were originally seen in an inpatient context. Second, client progress and the quality of the relationship as measured by the Session Rating Scale (SRS) covaried. Specifically, SRS scores generally improved over time for those in the successful group while remaining stable (whether beginning high or low) among the unsuccessful. Third, no difference in initial SRS scores was found between clients who made progress over the course of care and dropped out, deteriorated, or did not improve. Janice knew this was a potential target for DP, given evidence showing lower initial relationship ratings are associated with better results at the end of treatment (Miller et al., 2020). Fourth and finally, the modal number of sessions Janice had with clients was 1, with 32% attending only a single visit.

As a professional whose identity was closely tied to her commitment to excellence, Janice's performance data evoked both anxiety and a strong sense of inadequacy. On the recommendation of her supervisor/coach, she chose to spend the next month engaging in Exercise 2 (i.e., recovering your "university days" mindset). While she was typically focused on achievement and performance, she worked at being open to growth instead of just competence (Chow, 2019b). Although the change in mindset did not come easily, spending time with her performance data was what did the trick. She marveled at how the routine administration of simple measures could reveal patterns that had, despite her best intentions, eluded detection.

Eager to begin actively taking steps to address the problems identified, she returned to Exercise 3, determined to choose a single, committed outcome goal on which to work. Once again, Janice found herself struggling. Turns out, consultation with her supervisor/coach revealed the issue. It is a common one: focusing on the "how" before being clear about and committed to the "what." For example, given the various patterns her SRS data revealed, she decided to work on developing skills related to eliciting more detailed, critical feedback (TDPA Dimension 1A). She further concluded that adding more organization and focus to her sessions (TDPA Dimension 1J) would improve results with clients she initially met in an inpatient setting and treated for longer periods.

Returning to her spreadsheet to revisit the patterns and choose a single, committed outcome proved to be the solution. After recording the four patterns in her journal, Janice spent a week thinking about the clients with whom she had been unsuccessful, reviewing the case notes for each:

- Clients starting in an inpatient context (~65%) routinely failed to follow through with scheduled outpatient appointments.

- Clients whose SRS scores did not improve over the course of care were significantly more likely to end treatment with little or no improvement in Outcome Rating Scale scores.

- Clients with high initial SRS scores were equally likely to end treatment unsuccessfully as successfully.

- Nearly a third of Janice's clients did not return following their first session.

With help from her supervisor/coach, Janice chose what she believed would be the easiest to address. In this instance, that "low-hanging fruit" was the high number of unplanned terminations by clients first seen in an inpatient setting. Stated specifically, her outcome goal was to reduce dropouts for clients transitioning from inpatient to outpatient from 65% to 40%. The remaining three performance concerns were labeled "aspirational" and set aside for possible DP in the future.

Exercise 4 came next—figuring out the process goal that would decrease the dropout rate of inpatient clients. After watching video recordings of several representative sessions together with her supervisor/coach, both agreed the conversations conducted with hospitalized clients were more unfocused than typical outpatient visits. Consistent with Janice's lower rating on TDPA Dimension 3Ai (3/10), this led to the formulation of a process goal and learning project organized around establishing and checking goal consensus in first and later sessions. However, when Janice subsequently interviewed several former clients, a different angle emerged. A number mentioned being surprised by her questions about and characterization of not continuing with sessions on an outpatient basis as "dropping out."

Discussing her findings with her supervisor/coach, the two agreed hope and expectancy factors were implicated, one element of which (TDPA Dimension 2A & D regarding role induction, setting and monitoring client expectations, and adapting the treatment rationale to foster engagement and hope) Janice had also rated low (3/10) on her initial completion of the tool.

Janice immediately went to work creating a learning project, taking time to brainstorm, talk with colleagues, and research ideas related to operationalizing her process goal. Because she found clients frequently struggled to parlay improvements made while in the hospital to their lives following discharge, she created what she later termed her "safety-net" system. Introduced early in care, it emphasized the critical role she would play and resources she could bring to bear in supporting lasting change for the client. Appointment reminders and help with arranging transportation to and from sessions were two among the many aspects of the system specifically designed to reduce dropouts.

Together with her supervisor/coach, Janice continued to monitor her performance data as she put her plans into action. Six months later, she was disappointed when improvement in the percentage of clients failing to follow through with posthospitalization outpatient sessions stalled at 50%. At one point, she began actively considering replacing her committed outcome goals with one of her remaining (three) aspirational goals. "Actually," she said, "nearly all of the items on the TDPA are things I could work on and do better at. How can I *not* try to improve on more of these?"

Completing the "antigoal" exercise (5) persuaded Janice to maintain her current objective but reconsider her process goal. Addressing TDPA Factor 2 (hopes, expectations, and role) had resulted in a decline in dropouts, but she was looking for more. Returning to recordings of her sessions and consulting the therapy blueprint she had created at the outset of her foray into DP, she noted the significant amount of time spent in initial visits conducting a thorough psychosocial history. It was an activity that had been ingrained in her clinical routine from her university days—and yet, she realized, the information gathered only rarely informed her work, delayed actively intervening to help clients, and often resulted in lower levels of engagement.

At this time, she ran across the book *The First Kiss* (Chow, 2018), which focused on the importance of the initial therapeutic encounters. In place of "taking" (paperwork, information gathering, long diagnostic workups), it encouraged therapists "giving" to clients, taking full advantage of the change research shows occurs early in treatment (Lutz et al., 2009, 2014). The same body of evidence reviewed in the book showed traditional "intake" practices resulted in higher dropout rates, slower progress, and more expensive care. It also identified an alternative: *resource activation* (Gassmann & Grawe, 2006). Instead of asking about the presenting problem, symptoms, and struggles, it involves actively soliciting information about client capabilities, motivations, and existing social support network.

At this point, Janice made a conscious choice to change her process goal from Items A and D on Dimension 2 (relationship factors) of the TDPA to Dimension 4 (client factors), specifically, Item D, "incorporating your client's strengths, abilities, and resources into care." In support of this new objective, she sought out research, training materials, and consultation. After several months, Janice's hard work began to pay off. Interestingly, her discontinuation rates among those clients beginning care in an inpatient setting declined (from 50% to 18%), and the modal number of sessions she met with clients tripled (from 1 to 3). As often happens, such improvements influenced other performance metrics, including a rise in Janice's overall effectiveness (i.e., effect size).

FINAL CONSIDERATIONS

Our empathic disposition primes us to zoom in on one person rather than many. In so doing, developmental psychologist Paul Bloom (2016) argued, we become biased by the spotlight effect, missing bigger patterns, the so-called forest for the trees. The purpose of this chapter has been to marry our empathic ability with the systematic approach needed for successful DP. Whatever one's primary disposition, the process is hard work. Some suggestions born of experience follow:

- Unless your data indicate deficits in the structural domain of the TDPA, limiting your process goals and learning project to mastering a specific theoretical orientation is a mistake. Instead of aiming at "doing things right," focus on finding the "right thing" to improve your results. In other words, keep your eyes on the outcome goal.

- If the TDPA and OPL framework took you an hour or so to complete, it probably isn't going to serve you well. More time—much more time—is required.

- If your process goal feels easy, it's unlikely to stretch you sufficiently to improve your performance.

- If you are struggling with your process goal and learning project, your outcome goal may be too vaguely defined or ambitious.

- If your outcome goal is proving too difficult to achieve, designate it as "aspirational" and move on.

- If you find yourself losing track of what you were working on, consider reviewing your journal (i.e., notes) more often and making your learning project more visible.

- If your learning project and process goal are not leading to improvement in your outcome goal, consider the following:
  - whether your process goal is clearly linked to your outcome goal
  - allowing more time to pass before assessing results
  - whether adequate effort has been devoted to your process goal and learning project
  - consulting a coach

- Keep in mind that outcome goals do not always equate with improving or learning therapy skills. A high "no-show" rate, for example, might best be addressed by adopting an automated email or message reminder system rather than new engagement techniques or abilities (Martin et al., 2015).

DECISION POINT

What to do next:

- If you have completed the TDPA and OPL framework and need guidance developing an exercise for your specific objective, turn to
  - Chapter 3 for client factors
  - Chapter 4 for therapist factors
  - Chapter 5 for relationship factors
  - Chapter 6 for hope and expectancy factors
  - Chapter 7 for structure

- If you have used the TDPA to establish a specific, individualized learning objective but are struggling to stay focused or motivated, turn to Chapter 8.

REFERENCES

Agarwal, P. K., & Bain, P. M. (2019). *Powerful teaching: Unleash the science of learning.* Jossey Bass. https://doi.org/10.1002/9781119549031

Ahrens, S. (2017). *How to take smart notes: One simple technique to boost writing, learning and thinking—for students, academics and nonfiction book writers.* CreateSpace Independent Publishing Platform.

Bjork, R. A. (2011). On the symbiosis of remembering, forgetting, and learning. In A. S. Benjamin (Ed.), *Successful remembering and successful forgetting: A festschrift in honor of Robert A. Bjork* (pp. 1–22). Psychology Press.

Bloom, P. (2016). *Against empathy: The case for rational compassion.* HarperCollins.

Chow, D. (2014). *The study of supershrinks: Development and deliberate practices of highly effective psychotherapists* [Doctoral dissertation, Curtin University]. https://www.academia.edu/9355521/The_Study_of_Supershrinks_Development_and_Deliberate_Practices_of_Highly_Effective_Psychotherapists_PhD_Dissertation_

Chow, D. (2018). *The first kiss: Undoing the intake model and igniting first sessions in psychotherapy.* Correlate Press.

Chow, D. (2019a). *Deep learner: A psychotherapist's field guide to extend your mind and harness wisdom into clinical practice.* https://darylchowcourses.teachable.com/p/deeplearner

Chow, D. (2019b, October 22). Measure growth, not competence. *Frontiers of Psychotherapist Development.* https://darylchow.com/frontiers/measure-growth-not-competence

Chow, D., & Miller, S. D. (2022). *Taxonomy of Deliberate Practice Activities in Psychotherapy—Therapist Version* (Version 6). International Center for Clinical Excellence.

Chow, D. L., Miller, S. D., Seidel, J. A., Kane, R. T., Thornton, J. A., & Andrews, W. P. (2015). The role of deliberate practice in the development of highly effective psychotherapists. *Psychotherapy, 52*(3), 337–345. https://doi.org/10.1037/pst0000015

Doerr, J. (2018). *Measure what matters: OKRs—the simple idea that drives 10x growth.* Portfolio Penguin.

Gan, M., & Chen, S. (2017). Being your actual or ideal self? What it means to feel authentic in a relationship. *Personality and Social Psychology Bulletin, 43*(4), 465–478. https://doi.org/10.1177/0146167216688211

Gassmann, D., & Grawe, K. (2006). General change mechanisms: The relation between problem activation and resource activation in successful and unsuccessful therapeutic interactions. *Clinical Psychology & Psychotherapy, 13*(1), 1–11. https://doi.org/10.1002/cpp.442

Germer, S., Weyrich, V., Bräscher, A.-K., Mütze, K., & Witthöft, M. (2022). Does practice really make perfect? A longitudinal analysis of the relationship between therapist experience and therapy outcome: A replication of Goldberg, Rousmaniere, et al. (2016). *Journal of Counseling Psychology, 69*(5), 745–754. https://doi.org/10.1037/cou0000608

Goldberg, S. B., Rousmaniere, T., Miller, S. D., Whipple, J., Nielsen, S. L., Hoyt, W. T., & Wampold, B. E. (2016). Do psychotherapists improve with time and experience? A longitudinal analysis of outcomes in a clinical setting. *Journal of Counseling Psychology, 63*(1), 1–11. https://doi.org/10.1037/cou0000131

Haskell, R. E. (2001). *Transfer of learning: Cognition, instruction, and reasoning.* Academic Press. https://doi.org/10.1016/B978-012330595-4/50003-2

Klein, K., & Boals, A. (2001). Expressive writing can increase working memory capacity. *Journal of Experimental Psychology: General, 130*(3), 520–533. https://doi.org/10.1037/0096-3445.130.3.520

Lin, X., Miller, S. D., Chow, D., Goodyear, R., & Yang, A. (2022). *Return to Lake Wobegon: A cross-cultural replication of Walfish et al. (2012) and Chow et al. (2015)* [Manuscript in preparation]. Hubei Oriental Insight Mental Health Institute, China.

Lutz, W., Hofmann, S. G., Rubel, J., Boswell, J. F., Shear, M. K., Gorman, J. M., Woods, S. W., & Barlow, D. H. (2014). Patterns of early change and their relationship to outcome and early treatment termination in patients with panic disorder. *Journal of Consulting and Clinical Psychology, 82*(2), 287–297. https://doi.org/10.1037/a0035535

Lutz, W., Stulz, N., & Köck, K. (2009). Patterns of early change and their relationship to outcome and follow-up among patients with major depressive disorders. *Journal of Affective Disorders, 118*(1–3), 60–68. https://doi.org/10.1016/j.jad.2009.01.019

Martin, S. J., Goldstein, N. J., & Cialdini, R. B. (2015). *The small big: Small changes that spark big influence.* Profile Books.

Mathieu, F., Hubble, M., & Miller, S. D. (2015, May/June). Burnout reconsidered: What supershrinks can teach us. *Psychotherapy Networker.* https://www.psychotherapynetworker.org/magazine/article/36/burnout-reconsidered

McChesney, C., Covey, S., & Huling, J. (2012). *The 4 disciplines of execution.* Simon & Schuster.

Miller, S. D., Hubble, M., & Chow, D. (2018). The question of expertise in psychotherapy. *Journal of Expertise, 1*(2), 1–9.

Miller, S. D., Hubble, M., & Chow, D. (2020). *Better results: Using deliberate practice to improve therapeutic effectiveness.* American Psychological Association. https://doi.org/10.1037/0000191-000

Orlinsky, D. E., & Rønnestad, M. H. (2005). *How psychotherapists develop: A study of therapeutic work and professional growth.* American Psychological Association. https://doi.org/10.1037/11157-000

The University of Tulsa. (2020, November 5). *Normalizing the norm of changing college majors.* https://utulsa.edu/normalizing-the-norm-of-changing-college-majors/

Walfish, S., McAlister, B., O'Donnell, P., & Lambert, M. J. (2012). An investigation of self-assessment bias in mental health providers. *Psychological Reports, 110*(2), 639–644. https://doi.org/10.2466/02.07.17.PR0.110.2.639-644

3

Client Factors

Joshua K. Swift, Jesse Owen, and Scott D. Miller

Who should get the credit for this success? Foremost, of course, the patient.
— SÁNDOR FERENCZI,
THE CLINICAL DIARY OF SÁNDOR FERENCZI

DECISION POINT

Begin here if you have read the book *Better Results* and

- are routinely measuring your performance *and*
- have collected sufficient data to establish a reliable, evidence-based profile of your therapeutic effectiveness *and*
- have completed the Taxonomy of Deliberate Practice Activities in Psychotherapy *and*
- need help developing deliberate practice exercises which leverage client factors.

Imagine one day, a team of well-known theorists, researchers, and psychotherapists get together and, over the course of a year, develop a new treatment for depression. Excited about this new development, the team obtains grant funding and designs a rigorous randomized controlled trial to test the efficacy of the approach. They spare no expense in recruiting and screening participants, training study therapists, monitoring fidelity, and carrying out the study.

https://doi.org/10.1037/0000358-004
The Field Guide to Better Results: Evidence-Based Exercises to Improve Therapeutic Effectiveness,
S. D. Miller, D. Chow, S. Malins, and M. A. Hubble (Editors)

As the results are analyzed, they discover that 100% of the clients show clinically significant change. Even those who did not complete a full course of the treatment completely recovered by termination. Surprised by the results, the team conducts a second similar study, and again, 100% of the participants experienced clinically significant change. Other researchers begin testing the new treatment, and the results are always perfect—without exception, every person who receives it recovers!

Now, imagine we have a world-renowned psychotherapist who was part of the team who developed and tested the new approach. As expected, this clinician knows the treatment inside and out, has perfect mastery of it, and has now trained hundreds of others in its delivery. Then, one day, a client with depression presents for help. The "miracle" treatment is described, and on the basis of the existing research, the psychotherapist guarantees its success. However, the client is not interested. Because of their culture, values, and beliefs, they are not willing to engage in it. They understand the guarantee being made but choose to live with the depression rather than violate their principles and beliefs. So, while a 100% effective treatment delivered by an expert psychotherapist exists, the chance of it making a difference for this particular client is zero. The client—their willingness, motivation, culture, values, and preferences—is what determines the results of the treatment in this instance.

Although this scenario is presented in the extreme, a version of it plays out every day around the world. An experienced therapist, for example, may employ an evidence-based method (e.g., prolonged exposure therapy) while working with a veteran experiencing posttraumatic stress disorder (PTSD). However, the treatment does not seem to have an effect, and the client seems hesitant to engage fully. Through inquiry, the helper discovers that the accepted standard of care does not fit the client's explanation of their problems or the preferences they have for psychotherapy. In the client's mind, the PTSD reactions are closely linked to their strongly held spiritual beliefs and the guilt and moral injury they feel surrounding their combat experiences—something the research-supported treatment approach does not fully address.

As reviewed in detail in *Better Results* (*BR*; S. D. Miller et al., 2020), the evidence clearly shows psychotherapy is effective. That said, the effects are dependent on the individual client and how they engage and interact with the psychotherapist and the specific treatment approach applied (Wampold & Imel, 2015). Research over 5 decades makes clear that the contributions made by the client and extratherapeutic factors explain the majority of the variance in psychotherapy outcomes—greater than most other factors (e.g., the therapeutic relationship, the qualities of the therapist, hope and expectancy, and the technique or structure; Duncan et al., 2010; Hubble et al., 1999; Wampold & Imel, 2015).

Therefore, any therapist hoping to improve their effectiveness would increase their ability to work with and tailor their approach to the individual client. The material that follows provides a brief review of the evidentiary support for client factors, a distillation of evidence-based principles for accommodating and personalizing treatment to the client, and exercises therapists can employ in their deliberate practice (DP) to enhance their skills and competencies in this area.

REVIEW OF THE RESEARCH

In the following section, we review the research on the influence of client factors in psychotherapy. This includes a review of client factors that are known to exert little or no influence on treatment outcomes, as well as client factors that have been found to play an important role in psychotherapy.

Client Factors Exerting Little or No Influence on Outcomes

When asked to present a description of a particular client, it is not uncommon for clinicians to mention age, gender identity, sexual orientation, race, ethnicity, socioeconomic status, education level, and of course, diagnosis. These "client factors," so to speak, must therefore be considered relevant. As the first offered up for consideration, it is often assumed they are not only useful in providing a basic picture of who the client is but also important in informing care. Curiously, the evidence shows they play little to no role in determining the choice of treatment or its outcome.

Consider a recent and comprehensive review of the literature examining the link between client demographic characteristics (e.g., age, gender or gender identity, race or ethnicity, sexual orientation or identity, religiosity or spirituality, and socioeconomic status) and treatment outcomes conducted by Constantino et al. (2021). As can be seen in Table 3.1, evidence is either nonexistent, insufficient, mixed, or inconsistent.

TABLE 3.1. Summary of Research Findings on the Relationship Between Specific Client Demographic Factors, Treatment Outcome, and Dropout Rates

Demographic factor	Impact on outcome
Age	No significant or consistent correlation
Gender or gender identity	Inconsistent associations
	Insufficient research on nonbinary and transgender clients
	Within therapist disparities in outcomes
Race or ethnicity	Disparities in access and quality of care
	No significant or consistent correlation
	Within therapist disparities in outcomes
Sexual orientation	Insufficient
	Within therapist disparities in outcomes
Religion or spirituality	No significant or consistent correlation
Socioeconomic status	Limited evidence of poorer outcomes compared to higher socioeconomic status
	Small number of studies suggests caution when interpreting results

In all, Constantino and colleagues' (2021) review suggests practitioners be exceedingly cautious in drawing firm conclusions about the relationship between any single client demographic factor and psychotherapy outcome or dropout rate. Given the potential for bias, the state of the evidence calls into question the common practice of citing such variables in clinical discussions and notes or attempting to match clients to therapists or treatments based on such considerations alone (Cabral & Smith, 2011; Constantino et al., 2021). Indeed, with regard to the latter, the practice is deeply flawed. Matching therapist to client on the basis of individual demographic variables alone does not improve engagement or outcome (e.g., clients matched to therapists because they share the same gender, cultural identity, or sexual orientation; Cabral & Smith, 2011; Constantino et al., 2021).

Instead, an emerging line of research points to possibly a better way. This research suggests that the impact of specific demographic factors on outcome depends on *who* treats the client. Said another way, the relationship between therapeutic effectiveness and the race or ethnicity, sexual orientation, religious affiliation, and gender identity of clients is greater for some therapists than others (Budge & Moradi, 2018; Drinane et al., 2016, 2022; Hayes et al., 2015, 2016; Imel et al., 2011; Larrison et al., 2011; Owen et al., 2009, 2012, 2017). Imel et al. (2011), for instance, found that therapists differed significantly in their effectiveness depending on their clients' racial or ethnic makeup.

It is important to note research does show that clients—in particular, those belonging to a minority group—often prefer working with therapists similar to themselves (Cabral & Smith, 2011; Constantino et al., 2021; Swift et al., 2015). While this finding may, at first blush, appear to contradict earlier results documenting no clear relationship between outcome and client demographic factors, understanding how research on demographic variables is typically conducted provides clarification. Such studies are generally carried out at a group versus individual level, with all clients added together and the average reported. In so doing, individual differences (critical in the actual psychotherapy room) disappear. Matching could be, and often is, important to one client but not to all people with a similar quality, trait, background, or identity. Thus, the emphasis should be placed on the individual's preferences and values rather than on the group to which they belong.

While on the subject of matching, mention should be made of recent efforts to link treatment approaches to diagnosis. The "empirically supported treatment" movement, as it is called, seeks to identify specific psychological approaches for particular populations, groups, or disorders (Chambless & Hollon, 1998). While the commonsense appeal for therapists and clients is undeniable—especially in medicalized Western countries—research has not shown implementation to result in improved outcomes (Wampold & Imel, 2015). Even studies that have attempted to match clients to treatments along several demographic and psychological dimensions have failed to make a difference (e.g., Project MATCH, 1997). Known as the "ecological fallacy," the flaw, once again, is making inferences about individuals based on aggregated group data. More-over, focusing on demographic variables that do not have a direct influence on treatment outcomes may lead clinicians to overlook the client factors that do (i.e., client strengths, abilities, values, and beliefs as seen in the client factors section of the Taxonomy of Deliberate Practice Activities in Psychotherapy [TDPA; Chow & Miller, 2022; see Appendix A, this volume]).

Bottom line? Therapists maximize the chances of success by recognizing their clients as individuals rather than making assumptions about them based on qualities believed shared by the demographic group to which they belong. After all, demographic variables are simply labels. They do not capture the multidimensional nature of clients' various identities. After reviewing 50 years of Nigrescence, Cross (2021) noted, for example, the term "African American" collapses complex and diverse peoples in the United States into a single mono-lithic group (Cross, 2021). Rarely is the intersection of multiple client identities or the ones clients deem most salient to their life employed in studies of demo-graphic variables (Drinane et al., 2022; Hook et al., 2013; Owen, 2013).

To that end, consistent with the approach described in this volume and *BR* (S. D. Miller et al., 2020), a more helpful approach to addressing client demo-graphic factors includes therapists (a) formally and systematically monitoring their work; (b) analyzing the resulting data to determine which, if any, client demographic factors are reliably associated with less effective results on their part; and (c) targeting their professional development efforts at addressing any identified disparities in their ability to engage and help. After all, as is reviewed in the next section, research shows adapting care to clients' race or ethnicity, religion or spirituality has positive effects on treatment outcomes for some clients (Constantino et al., 2021; Huey et al., 2014; Soto et al., 2018).

Client Factors That Do Make a Difference

While the foregoing makes clear that treatment decisions should not be made based on a client's group membership, tailoring treatment to an *individual's* identity, values, and preferences is an important part of evidence-based practice in psychology (American Psychological Association Presidential Task Force on Evidence-Based Practice, 2006). As the factors that do make a difference are reviewed, it is important to keep in mind they are to be considered with a view toward tailoring and personalization. Take client preferences. Despite research showing that 75% of people with mental health concerns prefer psychotherapy over medication (McHugh et al., 2013), it would be wrong to assign all clients to psychotherapy first on the basis of the predilections of the majority. As we discussed for the demographic variables earlier, assump-tions about individual clients should not be made based on group findings and averages. Instead, each client needs to be asked about their particular prefer-ences and accommodated accordingly. The following variables emphasize the importance of tailoring to the individual client.

Role Expectations

Role expectations refer to clients' beliefs about what is likely to happen in treatment (Arnkoff et al., 2002), including the provider they might work with (e.g., gender, discipline, cultural background), what the treatment will look like (e.g., passive vs. active, daily vs. weekly visits), the roles the client and therapist will play (e.g., active vs. passive, directive vs. nondirective), and even how long a course of care might last (e.g., brief, intermittent, ongoing). Such beliefs can be based on past psychotherapy experiences, stereotypes played out in the media, or messages heard from friends and family. For example, because of portrayals in the movies, a client may believe they will be asked to lie on a couch. Alternatively, after talking to a family member about their experience in treatment, a client may believe their therapist will offer advice, giving detailed and explicit instructions for how to solve their problem. Client beliefs about psychotherapy can be accurate or faulty. For example, research indicates that most expect to attend fewer sessions than the evidence indicates are necessary to be effective (Bohart & Wade, 2013; Garfield, 1994; Swift & Callahan, 2008). As therapists vary in training, discipline, style, and approach, the fit between expectation and experience will also depend on who the client happens to meet.

Previous reviews of the literature have questioned the connection between role expectations and treatment outcome (Arnkoff et al., 2002). However, as was the case with research on demographic factors, the failure may say as much about the design of the studies as it does about their influence on outcome. It is possible, for example, that the negative effects of unmet role expectations for some clients are canceled out by the positive effects of met role expectations for others in the current summaries of the evidence.

What can be said with certainty is positive outcomes often follow when therapists spend time preparing their clients for what will happen. Known as "role induction" or "pretherapy education," this includes providing a rationale for what is being offered, a step-by-step outline of what will take place, and an explication of the role and expectations of the client in the process. Consider the evidence. Using data from 28 independent studies, a meta-analysis by Monks (1996) found that including some type of role induction at the start or before the beginning of psychotherapy led to increased treatment attendance ($d = 0.32$), decreased dropout ($d = 0.23$), and improved outcomes ($d = 0.34$), all with small to medium effects observed. In a second and more recent meta-analysis focused on strategies for increasing treatment attendance, data from 14 randomized controlled studies of pretreatment education showed a medium-size effect ($d = 0.50$) on attendance and decreasing dropout (Oldham et al., 2012). Similar results have been reported in studies testing strategies for addressing clients' role expectations concerning treatment duration. In the most often cited, Swift and Callahan (2011) found clients who received pretreatment education about adequate doses of psychotherapy attended nearly twice the number of sessions ($d = 0.55$) and were 3.5 times more likely to be classified as completers than clients who did not receive the educational preparation.

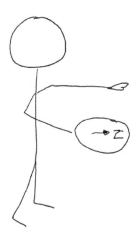

FIELD GUIDE TIP

Early on in *BR*, you were asked to create a schematic or blueprint for how you conduct therapy sufficiently detailed so another practitioner could understand and replicate it—literally, "step into your shoes" and work how you work (Miller et al., 2020, p. 29). The purpose of the activity was to make it easy to pinpoint where to intervene as opportunities for improving your effectiveness are identified by analyzing your performance data.

If you have not yet completed a blueprint, turn to pages 18–20 in this volume for updated, step-by-step directions.

Next, with your completed blueprint in hand,

- ensure it includes a description of how you prepare clients for what will take place in treatment once it begins; and

- should "role-induction" or "pretherapy education" be absent, turn to the Client Factors section (the fourth domain) of the TDPA and complete the first two items (A and B).

Preferences

While expectations represent clients' beliefs about what might happen during psychotherapy, preferences can be thought of as their desires for what they would want to occur were the choice left up to them (Swift et al., 2018). Like role expectations, clients may have preferences about the therapist with whom they work (e.g., age, gender, religious background, lived experience), the type of treatment they want to receive (e.g., client-centered vs. cognitive behavioral, directive vs. nondirective), and the nature of the care (e.g., homework, therapist advice giving, exploration). Like role expectations, preferences may be based on past experiences in therapy. Nevertheless, they can also be influenced by clients' likes and dislikes derived from other relationships, as well as knowledge about themselves. While client preferences frequently line up with elements of care most likely to lead to treatment success (Tompkins et al., 2017), this is not always the case. The evidence shows, for example, that comfort rather than effectiveness may drive the desire for certain therapist attributes, treatments, or situations (Swift & Callahan, 2010).

Research documents a number of benefits associated with accommodating client preferences. A major meta-analysis (Swift et al., 2018) using data drawn from 53 studies found significantly larger gains in posttreatment outcomes ($d = 0.28$) for clients whose preferences were accommodated compared with those whose were not. Retention in treatment was also significantly affected, with those whose preferences went unmatched dropping out at a 50% higher rate. Such effects were consistent across client age, gender, ethnicity, and years of education and, in terms of impact on outcome, even larger for clients with anxiety or depression concerns. And finally, while perhaps not surprising, the evidence shows preference accommodation also leads to stronger ratings of the therapeutic alliance (Windle et al., 2020), a robust predictor of treatment outcomes (Flückiger et al., 2018; see also Chapter 5, this volume). Swift et al. (2021) argued persuasively that choice and a spirit of collaboration can be empowering to clients, encouraging them to invest more in the work to ensure their choices prove successful.

Motivation and Stages of Change

As all clinicians know, hope and expectation of success in treatment (see Chapter 6 for an in-depth review) do not always translate into clients being ready or willing to put in the effort required to make desired changes happen. A large body of literature shows treatment that fits the client's motivational level or "readiness" is associated with more engagement and better outcomes (Norcross et al., 2011). The findings are robust, with the latest meta-analysis—including data from 76 different studies (Krebs et al., 2018)—reporting a medium-size effect ($d = 0.41$) when therapists successfully tailor treatment to the client's "stage of change."

According to the stages of change model (Prochaska & DiClemente, 1983), client motivation or readiness for a particular type or intensity of intervention can be classified into one of six different categories: (a) precontemplation (little to no awareness a problem exists and hence, no intention or desire to change), (b) contemplation (aware a problem exists and weighing the costs and benefits of change), (c) preparation (getting ready to take steps to change), (d) action (actively taking steps to address a problem), (e) maintenance (actively working to maintain a change and prevent relapse), and (f) recurrence (dealing with a setback or relapse). As illustrated in Table 3.2, each stage is associated with change processes or interventions most likely to facilitate—or at least not serve as a barrier to—moving to the next (Krebs et al., 2018).

The key is tailoring the nature, type, and pace of the intervention (e.g., therapist activity) to fit each client's current state of readiness. So, for example, telling a client in precontemplation to "attend 90 AA meetings in 90 days" would likely arouse feelings of mistrust and misunderstanding and increase the chances of them dropping out of care, whereas empathizing with their situation and providing information related to their particular concerns or questions would enhance the chances of their returning for future sessions. However, for a client in the action stage, mere listening and empathizing would likely lead to feelings of frustration with the pace of treatment. It must be emphasized that working at being "in sync" with where clients are is an ongoing process, critical throughout treatment as decisions are made about the various interventions.

TABLE 3.2. The Stages of Change, Associated Change Processes, and Congruent Stage-Specific Therapeutic Interventions

Stage of change	Change process	Intervention
Precontemplation (not seeing a problem or need for change)	Establishing rapport Building trust and connection Securing engagement Raising awareness	Listening Empathizing Being nonjudgmental Providing information about topics and options of interest to the client Using harm reduction strategies
Contemplation (thinking about changing)	Addressing ambivalence and uncertainty Evaluating current behavior and outcomes Assessing and exploring client self-efficacy	Exploring specific options Weighing costs and benefits of change Modeling and exploring what changing looks like Connecting with people who support making a change
Preparation (planning to make a change)	Establishing objectives Organizing efforts Securing necessary resources and supports	Setting goals Planning Establishing timelines Identifying helpful supports and resources Considering potential barriers to success Offering practical help, support, and positive reinforcement
Action (taking steps)	Providing valuation and feedback Providing refinement Providing support	Monitoring successes and failures Identifying high risk and high success situations Using counterconditioning Managing reinforcement Providing coaching and advice
Maintenance (ensuring stable change)	Supporting, affirming, reinforcing Reviewing long-term goals and objectives	Providing stimulus control Providing coping strategies Finding connections with community of support
Recurrence	Learning from experience	Normalizing Providing feedback Providing support Reconnecting with supportive community

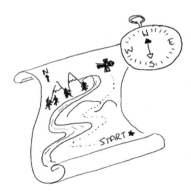

FIELD GUIDE TIP

"Stages of change," "change processes," and "interventions" provide a concrete, evidence-based illustration of Goldfried's (1980) "theoretical framework," "clinical strategies," and "techniques" described in Chapter 1 (p. 19).

Attachment Styles

Clients enter treatment with unique ways of relating to and interacting with the world and those around them. Research points to a link between what is commonly referred to in the literature as client "attachment styles" and the outcome of psychotherapy. In a meta-analysis of 32 studies, for example, Levy et al. (2018) found a moderate ($d = 0.35$) relationship. Specifically, higher levels of attachment security in clients at the outset of care were associated with more positive outcomes at termination.

However impressive such findings may appear at first blush, results of studies examining group-level differences, as previously discussed, are not particularly applicable to conducting therapy with an individual. They might, were therapists able to limit their work to clients with the same attachment style! Given therapists are typically unable to choose the starting attachment style of their clients, adjusting services to fit each, once therapy starts, is wise. To that end, Table 3.3 presents the four main attachment styles, associated

TABLE 3.3. Attachment Style, Style Characteristics, and Prevalence

Attachment style	Characteristics	Prevalence
Secure	Able to easily and quickly form secure, loving relationships with others Trusting and trustworthy Loving and lovable	50% to 60% of adults
Anxious	Insecure about relationships Fearful of abandonment Hungry for validation	15% to 25% of adults
Avoidant	Insecure and distant in relationships Emotionally unavailable Independent and self-reliant Has difficulty being close with or trusting others	20% to 30% of adults
Fearful–avoidant	Combination of the anxious and avoidant styles Craves and avoids affection and intimacy	Less researched, but believed rare

characteristics, and prevalence. Importantly, research suggests changes in attachment can occur in psychotherapy and are associated with positive outcomes. In their meta-analysis, for example, Levy and colleagues (2018) found movement toward attachment security during treatment led to better outcomes ($r = .16$), while lowering levels of attachment anxiety was linked with greater improvements in both symptoms ($r = .18$) and functioning ($r = .16$). In addition, lower levels of attachment avoidance were associated with greater improvements in symptoms ($r = .15$).

Reactance

Reactance has been identified as an emotional reaction that people have when they feel that their ability to make a choice is being threatened (Brehm & Brehm, 1981). This reaction often leads to a stronger preference for the options that are perceived as being limited or taken away. Research shows higher levels of reactance are associated with a greater likelihood of rejecting and derogating health-promoting messages and their sources (e.g., health care professionals; C. H. Miller et al., 2007). Fortunately, the same body of literature shows reactance levels are influenceable. C. H. Miller et al. (2007), for example, found concrete (vs. abstract), low-controlling communication, emphasizing the choices available to the listener, were viewed as more important, received more attention, and generated more positive assessments of the source.

As all clinicians know, psychotherapy can be difficult for clients. It may require them to approach thoughts, memories, feelings, and situations they have previously labored to avoid. Alternately, change may require giving up habits, coping styles, and even personal relationships, previously comforting or rewarding. Not surprisingly, this may give rise to reactance in which, consciously or unconsciously, the client opposes the change process (Brehm & Brehm, 1981). Like the findings reported in the broader health care literature, research shows the degree of reactance can be influenced by the therapist's approach. Consider a recent meta-analysis by Beutler et al. (2018) synthesizing data from 13 different studies. It found a large effect ($d = 0.79$) when treatment was tailored to the level of client reactance. Specifically, outcomes were significantly better when therapists of highly reactive clients assumed a less directive, more reflective stance. By contrast, clients low in reactance fared better when therapists were more active and directive in treatment. Clearly, adjusting services to fit client reactance level is a potent way to improve client engagement and outcome. It is consistent with the "mobilization of will" listed in the relationship factors dimension of the TDPA and, when framed as a positive client trait, can also be seen as a way of tapping into clients' strengths, values, and abilities specified in the client factor domain.

Culture

Cultural adaptations, therapists' cultural competence, and therapist multicultural orientation are positively associated with treatment outcome. A recent meta-analysis by Soto and colleagues (2018) identified 99 studies of culturally adapted treatments and 15 addressing the link between therapist cultural competence and outcomes. Culturally adapted interventions were significantly more effective than nonadapted interventions for racial and ethnic minority clients (medium size, $d = 0.50$). Client ratings of their therapist's cultural competence were strongly correlated with effective treatment ($r = .38$). The same analysis indicated that higher client ratings of therapist multicultural orientation are associated with stronger alliances, which, in turn, lead to better results. Therapist ratings of their own cultural competence were, by contrast, *not* related to outcome. Like alliance-related findings (Horvath et al., 2011), it is the *client's* perception of their therapist's cultural awareness, knowledge, and skills that matters most, not the therapist's judgment of their own competence, sensitivity, or abilities.

Adapting care to each client's culture—a practice now known in the literature as *dynamic sizing*—is easier said than done (S. Sue, 2006). In truth, it is much like threading a needle, the challenge being promoting engagement while avoiding stereotyping. A case in point: Manualized therapies have been created for treating people with eating disorders. To be culturally sensitive, specific adaptations to the standardized protocols have been suggested regarding the types of foods to be discussed and included in treatment interventions (e.g., a "Mexican food guide for Latina women" presenting with bulimia; Reyes-Rodríguez et al., 2014). Other modifications include employing culturally specific stories and characters to shape or frame therapeutic interventions (Costantino et al., 1986). The danger, of course, is presuming everyone who shares a particular ethnicity eats the same foods or finds the same customs or concepts meaningful. People always look more similar from a distance, and yet, what is assumed to apply to the many may, in fact, not apply to any given person.

Beyond losing sight of individual differences, the sheer number of possible adaptations can quickly become unmanageable. Official definitions of multicultural competence already include being both aware of and accommodating differences in race, ethnicity, gender, sexual orientation, culture, religion, and spirituality. Once one adds, as is recommended, age, maturity, socioeconomic status, class standing, family history, and a host of other process and demographic variables, even the most conscientious of practitioners cannot help but be overwhelmed. To illustrate, in a course of psychotherapy, where a clinician considers only two of the 13 factors just identified, 78 possible adaptations to the treatment obtain. Add one and that number triples. If only four dimensions are identified as consequential, clinicians must master 715 different ways to nuance service delivery. Obviously, any standard of care that requires clinicians to juggle so many variables is both absurd and out of touch, with research showing people are incapable of multitasking (Atchley, 2010).

At length, were it possible to compile an exhaustive list of every cultural variable and therapists were somehow capable of managing all, a serious problem would remain. Unless the fundamental organizing principles and practices underlying clinical work are questioned, any accommodation, no matter how well-intentioned or comprehensive, risks being little more than window-dressing, a marketing hook, or the proverbial "spoonful of sugar" that makes the therapist's "medicine" more palatable. In place of what might be called the "chapter-in-a-book" approach to culture adaptation (e.g., do "X" with clients of African descent, do "Y" with Asian clients, and so on), Owen et al. (2011; Owen, 2013) offered what has been termed the "multicultural orientation framework," a way of being with clients rather than a predetermined approach for doing therapy. The multicultural orientation framework rests on three pillars: (a) cultural humility, (b) cultural opportunities, and (c) cultural comfort.

Being a humble therapist means having an accurate perception of one's own values—including the cultural assumptions informing or implicit in the methods employed—while simultaneously being able to maintain another, relationally oriented perspective that sponsors respect, equity, and connection (Davis et al., 2018; Fancher, 1995; Hook et al., 2013). In practice, this means working continuously on self-awareness (e.g., one's biases, strengths, weaknesses), bringing curiosity to every interaction, and being open to the client—especially feedback regarding the success achieved in understanding their experience and world. In addition, cultural humility is at the heart of understanding another's values and worldviews while reminding therapists to monitor their judgments. Studies to date demonstrate clients who view their therapist as more culturally humble have better therapy outcomes, including key therapeutic processes, such as the working alliance (e.g., Davis et al., 2018; Hook et al., 2013, 2016; Owen et al., 2014).

Seeking out and being responsive to cultural opportunities means being both aware of and willing to explore and integrate the intersection of clients' cultural heritage throughout the process of therapy (Owen, 2013; Owen et al., 2016). "Each therapy session provides multiple [such] opportunities," Hook et al. (2017) noted, "but for variety of reasons many of these . . . go unrealized" (p. 32). A simple example is ensuring that questions about culture on intake paperwork are broadly inclusive, reflecting a wide range of identities (e.g., open-ended vs. forced choice responses allowing clients to present who they are and what matters most to them). For clients, the evidence shows missing such opportunities results in poorer treatment outcomes (Owen et al., 2016).

Finally, cultural comfort refers to the feelings surrounding culturally relevant conversations in therapy. Discussing issues related to culture can be difficult and uncomfortable. Therapists with high levels of cultural comfort are able to manage their own feelings, engaging the client in a composed, relaxed, and connected manner. As a result, their clients are more likely to discuss cultural topics and form stronger therapeutic alliances (Tao et al., 2016). By contrast, racial and ethnic minority clients who meet with less "culturally comfortable" therapists are more likely to drop out of treatment (Owen et al., 2016).

Religion and Spirituality

Research clearly supports the integration of clients' religious and spiritual beliefs and practices into the process of psychotherapy. On the basis of data from 102 independent samples, one meta-analysis (Captari et al., 2018) found clients who received religious and spiritual tailoring showed more positive psychological and spiritual outcomes than those in control groups ($g = 0.75$ and $g = 0.75$, respectively) and nontailored treatment ($g = 0.33$ and $g = 0.43$, respectively). Not surprisingly, perhaps, the most rigorously designed studies in the analysis found standard treatments were as effective as tailored therapies in reducing psychological distress but significantly less effective in improving spiritual well-being ($g = 0.34$) and more positive psychological outcomes. The findings were consistent across client age, gender, presenting problem, and religious affiliation and even more effective for racial and ethnic minority clients.

Although therapists as a group remain less religious than those they serve, surveys consistently show most of their clients believe religion and spirituality are important and appropriate topics for psychotherapy (Miller & Hubble, 2017). In fact, most welcome questions and want to discuss their beliefs, viewing them as an integral part of their treatment experience (Dimmick et al., 2021; Martinez et al., 2007; Rose et al., 2001; Rosmarin et al., 2015). Unfortunately, Trusty et al. (2022) found that a sizeable number who consider themselves religious experience at least one *microaggression*—defined as subtle, denigrating comments or behaviors—during therapy, the most common being the minimization or avoidance of religious or spiritual issues.

Consistent with research findings on other client factors (e.g., culture or ethnicity), such experiences are negatively associated with the therapeutic alliance and outcome. Concrete and specific guidance for avoiding such missteps and integrating client spirituality and religion into psychological care can be found in a popular and widely read article, "How Psychotherapy Lost Its Magick," by Scott Miller and Mark Hubble (2017)—read more than 70,000 times at the time of the publication of the *Field Guide*. The authors presented a three-step framework, noting, "In some important ways, practitioners are already doing some of this work, but other aspects will undoubtedly prove more challenging, requiring a radical shift in the way psychotherapy is conceived and performed" (p. 33). From easiest to most challenging, the steps include

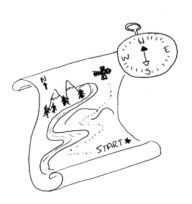

FIELD GUIDE TIP

Chapter 8 of *BR* describes and illustrates how to mine your performance data for deliberate practice opportunities. In light of the research presented in this section, consider sorting your clients according to their cultural, religious, or spiritual identity, paying particular attention to differences in alliance scores, dropout rates, and effect size.

(a) being willing to ask about and explore beliefs (exploration), (b) consciously and purposefully working to increase the fit between clients' religious and spiritual beliefs and the therapist's preferred way of thinking about and doing therapy (entering), and (c) using and incorporating religious practices (e.g., prayer, drumming, energy meridians) in care (embodying).

Sexual Orientation and Gender Identity

In recent years, some researchers have begun to develop and test lesbian, gay, bisexual, transgender, and queer (LGBTQ+)–affirmative therapies. As noted in the section on demographic variables, the number of studies in this area is insufficient to draw any firm conclusions regarding their potential advantage (Constantino et al., 2021). That said, two systematic reviews of the literature reported, like findings on other demographic variables, that the type of treatment is less important in terms of outcome and dropout than whether a therapist is open; curious; aware of their own preferences and biases; avoids subtle, denigrating comments or behaviors; and provides a safe, validating, and affirmative therapeutic environment (Budge & Moradi, 2018; Moradi & Budge, 2018). Transgender clients, in particular, express a strong desire for knowledgeable therapists and affirming therapies, having often experienced harm in psychotherapy resulting from clinicians' gender incompetence (Duffy et al., 2016; Elder, 2016). Given that therapists can err by either ignoring or overemphasizing gender identity or sexual orientation, the key—as with culture, religion, and spirituality—is being willing to explore connections between therapy and client sexual orientation or gender identity as guided by the individual client (Budge & Moradi, 2018).

Environmental Supports and Personal Strengths

A 2008 meta-analysis of 27 studies and more than 5,500 clients by Roehrle and Strouse reported a small but significant association ($r = .13$) between greater client social support—both perceived and extant—and psychotherapy outcome. While a handful of subsequent studies have returned more mixed results (e.g., Leibert et al., 2011), the weight of the evidence supports therapists routinely assessing the quantity and quality of actual supports, including the client's evaluation of their value and importance, and incorporating the findings in the conduct of therapy. For example, in their study, Leibert et al. (2011) showed an emphasis on the therapeutic alliance was particularly beneficial for clients with low social support. However, Project MATCH determined that the community provided by Alcoholics Anonymous proved more effective than comparison treatments for problem drinkers whose existing social network supported their alcohol use versus sobriety (Longabaugh et al., 1998).

Over the years, much has been written about the role of client strengths in psychotherapy. Indeed, entire models (e.g., solution-focused, positive psychology) have been developed on the basis of the premise that incorporating clients' strengths and abilities is a critical and overlooked key to success. While the number of clinical trials is low, one meta-analysis found no difference between strengths-based and other methods in either level of functioning or quality of life in adults diagnosed with severe mental illness (Ibrahim et al., 2014). Such findings are consistent with studies comparing different modalities, indicating it is not *the* treatment approach per se that matters but a question of *how* client strengths are approached within each session. Consider the results of two studies, both of which demonstrated a relationship between outcome and the timing and proportion of problem versus resource (e.g., strength) focus and discussion. Gassmann and Grawe (2006) explored the occurrence of problem and resource activation strategies in recordings of 120 sessions of psychotherapy drawn from a large sample of adult outpatient clients. Using a composite measure of outcome consisting of goal attainment, emotional, behavioral, and relational change and posttreatment client and therapist ratings, the researchers found (a) resource activation accounted for significantly more outcome variance than problem focus, and (b) a higher ratio of resource to problem activation differentiated successful from unsuccessful therapies.

Using multilevel modeling, Malins et al. (2021) showed specific types of therapeutic interactions predicted the experience of client well-being session by session; specifically, the greater the proportion of first and second sessions spent describing problems (as opposed to more active discussions of what to do with problems arising), the poorer the outcome. An analysis of therapeutic interactions with a smaller subset of clients ($n = 12$) revealed that time spent describing problems was much lower and positive discussions much higher in sessions immediately preceding client reports of rapid, sudden progress (see the discussion in the next section).

Taken together, the results just reported are consistent with Points D and F of the client factors dimension on the TDPA, emphasizing the possibilities inherent in assessing and using clients' existing strengths and social support networks.

Extratherapeutic Change-Producing Events

Researchers Howard et al. (1986) were the first to note, in their classic article, "The Dose-Effect Relationship in Psychotherapy," a sizeable number of clients (15%) were already experiencing improvement before the initial meeting with a therapist. Subsequent research suggests the incidence of pretreatment change is much higher—with as many as two thirds of clients reporting progress related to their reason for seeking help *if* the topic is raised for discussion by the therapist (Lawson, 1994; Reuterlov et al., 2000; Weiner-Davis et al., 1987). Other studies of adults and children have shown many experience significant therapeutic gains *early* in treatment that are both predictive of final treatment outcome and maintained at follow-up (Dour et al., 2013; Stiles et al., 2003; Tang & DeRubeis, 1999). In 2020, a meta-analysis of 50 studies by Shalom and Aderka found such "sudden gains" were highly predictive of outcome at termination ($g = 0.68$) and follow-up ($g = 0.61$), exceeding the variance attributable to specific treatments, diagnoses, and settings. Consistent with the recommendation in the client factors section of the TDPA, regardless of treatment approach or orientation, therapists should be open to, curious about, and welcoming of change wherever and whenever it occurs.

EVIDENCE-BASED PRINCIPLES RELATED TO CLIENT FACTORS

In presenting evidence-based principles related to client factors, one approach is to develop a comprehensive list of suggestions, each linking to one of the specific elements reviewed. For example, a list of principles could be offered for accommodating each client preference noted in the literature (e.g., offer clients the type of therapy they request, work at matching the client with a therapist who fits their particular preferences regarding age, gender, lived experience), followed by suggestions for religious and spiritual integration (e.g., create a list of specific practices to use with clients from specific religious backgrounds, develop therapeutic approaches incorporating the concepts and beliefs of specific religious), culture, and so on. In so doing, however, dozens of principles could be identified, each resulting in a long list of specific therapeutic "dos and don'ts" (for such a list, see Norcross & Wampold, 2018). While such an approach has the advantage of specificity, a more accurate representation of the findings in this area suggests a handful of principles applicable across all client factors reviewed in this chapter. Thus, regardless of who the client is, the following principles can be used to guide therapists in the development of DP exercises aimed at improving their ability to tailor their work to the individual client.

Principle 1: Treat Each Client as an Individual Rather Than a Member or Representative of a Particular Group (e.g., Demographic, Preference, Culture, Beliefs, or Diagnosis)

Some therapists may believe they are tailoring because, for example, they use a specific "culturally adapted" treatment for all their African American clients. Although this is a step in the right direction and will lead to outcomes across all their clients of African descent, it will misfire for many. As noted previously, group data does apply to individual clients. Some may desire cultural adaptations, others not. It is important that therapists not make assumptions about the individual based on how they look or the group with which they are identified. Similarly, it might be tempting, given the documented efficacy of religious and spiritual adaptations in psychotherapy, to include religious and spiritual discussions and techniques for any religious and spiritual client. Recall, however, existing research indicates some strongly religious individuals do *not* desire their beliefs to be a part of their psychotherapy (Dimmick et al., 2021), while many nonreligious individuals do (Rosmarin et al., 2015).

Principle 2: Actively Solicit Information About Each Client's Identity (e.g., Gender, Race and Ethnicity, Sexual Orientation, Religion and Spirituality) and Elements Known to Impact Psychotherapy Positively (e.g., Expectations, Preferences, Reactance, and Stage of Change)

When getting to know a client, interest should be on not only what their identities are but also how those intersect with their presenting problems and at what level they would like those identities discussed and incorporated into therapy. In so doing, it is important to remember such considerations might not always overlap for the individual. A highly religious client may link their psychological distress to religious concerns, for example, but may not want to include any religious or spiritual interventions or techniques in their psychotherapy. Rather, they may prefer to reserve any such approaches or discussions to religious settings and leaders. Alternatively, a different client may report no spiritual or religious distress but wish to end each session with a prayer.

With regard to expectations, preferences, and motivation, be mindful of what is available and possible in the treatment context. If only female clinicians are available at a particular agency, for example, asking whether the client had ideas about the type of therapist they would work best with is preferable to "Would you rather see a male or female?" Should a particular preference be unavailable, an opportunity can be offered to explore their reaction (e.g., feelings, thoughts), including the desire for a referral.

It is increasingly common for clients to express a preference for a particular brand or type of treatment (e.g., cognitive behavior therapy, eye movement desensitization and reprocessing therapy). Because such requests are tied to the client's reasons for seeking care, they should be encouraged and explored. Knowing a client believes their problems are biological in nature might lead to different engagement strategies (e.g., exercise, diet, medication) than if they viewed their concerns as primarily interpersonal in origin (e.g., relationship skills, assertiveness training, family therapy). In short, accommodating client preferences is more like a negotiation aimed at establishing a common understanding than ordering a meal from the menu of a restaurant (e.g., "Would you like your therapy with fries or a salad?").

Principle 3: Seek to Understand and Be Respectful of the Individual Client's Values and Beliefs, Even When They Are Different From the Ones Held by the Therapist

As reported earlier, when it comes to cultural and religious identity, a large percentage of clients report experiencing microaggressions from their therapists (e.g., 50%–75% of clients; Constantine, 2007; Hook et al., 2016; Owen et al., 2010, 2014; Shelton & Delgado-Romero, 2013; Trusty et al., 2022). To be sure, it is unlikely the majority of offenders intend to interact with certain clients in a hostile manner. Indeed, perpetrators typically find it difficult to believe they possess any biased attitudes whatsoever (D. W. Sue et al., 1992). Therefore, a good starting point for putting Principle 3 into practice would be to follow the ancient Greek aphorism "know thyself."

In terms of expectations, preferences, and motivation, differences in the values and beliefs between therapists and clients are also bound to occur. Consider, for example, the pairing of an active, task-oriented therapist with a depressed client who complains about homework suggestions. In such a case, attributing a lack of engagement or progress to "client resistance" would privilege the therapist's beliefs, values, and experience over the client's. A more effective approach, according to the research cited previously, would be to adjust the nature, type, and pace of intervention (e.g., therapist activity) to the client's state of readiness.

Some clients may have expectations regarding therapy that are inaccurate or uninformed. Therapists who immediately dismiss these types of expectations or preferences risk rupturing the therapeutic alliance. Balancing openness to the client's point of view with the provision of information is key for securing the engagement needed to derive a joint plan. For example, when asked about expected treatment duration, a client might reply they expect to recover fully in two sessions. In response, the therapist could recognize the client's initial expectation (e.g., "That is great! It sounds like you are optimistic about treatment and believe that it can help you quickly. Your optimism will be helpful as we work together"), provide information (e.g., "Although treatment might work that quickly for you, it typically doesn't work that fast for most people. In fact, the research suggests that it takes around 13 to 18 sessions for 50% of clients to recover. Some do recover sooner than that, but others take longer"), and develop a joint plan (e.g., "How about we plan on doing the first two sessions and then, at the end of the second session, we do a check-in to see where you are at. If things are all better at that point, that is great, and we will be done. But, if you need more than that, then we can plan for a few more sessions together until you get to where you want to be"). Understanding and respecting clients' values and beliefs is a concrete way to operationalize the TDPA client factor regarding values and beliefs while simultaneously making space for the therapist to better incorporate the client's strengths, abilities, and resources in treatment.

Principle 4: Check in With Clients on an Ongoing Basis to Ensure the Work Fits With Their Expectations, Preferences, Values, Needs, and Identity, Being Flexible and Accommodating When Needed

Clients' goals, desires, and expectations change and evolve while in therapy. What they thought they wanted at the outset may not be what they actually want once they see it in practice! Circumstances in clients' lives outside of therapy may also change. Consider someone who initially presents for help with work-related stress but learns her partner is having an affair and intends to end their relationship. Frequent "check-ins" allow therapists to identify and respond to shifts in goals, preferences, and alliance ruptures before clients choose to drop out (Swift & Greenberg, 2015). Using brief end-of-session measures such as the Session Rating Scale (described in detail in *BR*) is a particularly helpful way to ensure the therapy and therapist evolves *with* the client. It also provides a concrete method for identifying and incorporating client strengths and abilities, social support, and chance events into care, consistent with the recommendations on the TDPA.

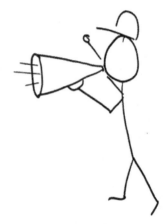

FIELD GUIDE TIP

"Certain therapists are *more* effective than others . . . because [they are] appropriately responsive . . . providing each client with a different, individually tailored treatment" (Stiles & Horvath, 2017, p. 71).

EXERCISES FOR CLIENT FACTOR SKILL DEVELOPMENT

While considering the following exercises, recall that "the goal of DP is neither proficiency nor mastery. Rather, it is all about continuously reaching for objectives that lie just beyond one's current ability" (Chapter 1, this volume). Said another way, no benefit will result from picking an exercise or two from the following list to engage in during your free time. To make a difference in your results, the exercise you choose must be specifically remedial to data-identified deficits in your clinical performance. As stated at the outset of this chapter, it is assumed you (a) are routinely measuring your performance; (b) have collected sufficient data to establish a reliable, evidence-based profile of your therapeutic effectiveness; (c) completed the TDPA; (d) determined a deficit exists in your performance related to the operation of client factors; and (e) narrowed your focus to a single element within the client factors domain on the TDPA and defined that performance improvement objective in SMART terms (specific, measurable, achievable, relevant, and time bound).

Now, with the completed TDPA in hand, review the following exercises for the one most closely aligned with your goal. Keep in mind the list is neither comprehensive nor exhaustive. You may, along with colleagues or peers, have ideas of your own. Should none of the exercises speak directly to your needs, Chapter 2 may prove helpful. It describes a process for using the TDPA in combination with your data to develop a "learning project," ultimately resulting in individualized DP exercises.

Exercise 1: Alternative Descriptions

Principle: 1
Applicability: TDPA Items 4C, E, F (also applicable to 3Bi, ii, iii, v, 5Aii, iv, 5Bi)
Purpose
When speaking about our clients to other providers, we often describe them based on their disorder or basic demographic variables (e.g., age, gender, ethnicity, sexual orientation). Although such descriptors allow for quick and

easy communication, they may result in erroneous, simplistic, or stereotypical assumptions. This exercise is designed to help therapists develop their skills in making individual decisions about clients rather than on group assumptions (either assumptions based on the empirical literature in the field or assumptions based on individual biases).

Task

Identify clients who have dropped out, reported low or declining scores on the alliance measure you routinely administer at the end of each visit (e.g., Session Rating Scale), or whose outcomes are either not improving or declining (e.g., Outcome Rating Scale). Using paper and pencil, word processing software, or your favorite note-keeping app, begin writing a brief description of each, focusing specifically on who they are as individuals rather than how they are similar to other clients. The "Four S" approach (Chow, 2022) may be helpful in completing the process, noting their *sense of self* (e.g., beliefs, personality, what they identify with), *sparks* (e.g., what they care about, what makes them come alive), *significant life events* (e.g., traumas, fortuitous and formulative happenings), and *systems* (e.g., positive and negative impactful relationships, critical environmental supports). Take your time in completing the task. Devoting a few minutes each day to the exercise is likely to prove more helpful in fostering the thinking and reflecting necessary to have an impact on subsequent performance than trying to complete it in a single sitting.

To the description, now add a case conceptualization. Do so without mentioning a specific psychiatric diagnosis or disorder, presenting problem, demographic characteristic, or another descriptor typically associated with clinically oriented presentations. Continue this process with new and existing clients when they meet the previously noted criteria.

After a month, or once a sufficient number of such descriptions and case conceptualizations have accumulated (~10–20), review and reflect on what you have written. Look for patterns. Return to the research review or recommended readings section of the chapter for ideas about expanding the ways you view and interact with clients. When not doing psychotherapy, take time to develop concrete examples (e.g., by writing out, role-playing) of including such ideas in your daily work.

Exercise 2: Asking About Preferences

Principle: 2
Applicability: TDPA Items 4A, B, C, E (also applicable to 3Bi, ii, v; 3Ci)
Purpose
Treatment decisions are guided by therapist beliefs, values, and preferences. The following exercise is designed to help therapists identify and then use client preferences to inform and enhance clinical decision making.

Tasks
Retrieve the schematic or blueprint you created for how to do therapy as described on page 29 of *BR* and updated in Chapter 1 in the *Field Guide*

(pp. 18–20). If exploring and accommodating client beliefs, values, and preferences at the outset of care are not specifically mentioned, add them to your map. Include a detailed description of what you talk over explicitly with your clients and how.

Next, note the beliefs, values, and preferences reviewed in the research section of this chapter that are not included in your map or usual way of working. Using paper and pencil, word processing software, or your favorite note-keeping app, write out how you would initiate a conversation with clients about those particular values and beliefs. For example, if clients' prior treatment experience was not a topic you typically asked about or explored, you would write out an initial question (i.e., "I would like to hear about your past experiences, if any, in psychotherapy"), along with several ways to follow up (i.e., "What went well?" "What didn't go so well?" "On the basis of these experiences, what would you want our work together to look like?"). With a client who has no prior experience in psychotherapy, you could ask, "Before coming in for our appointment today, did you have any thoughts about what you would like to happen as we work together?" following up with, "Did you have any worries about things I might do that you really do not want to be a part of your treatment?"

Complete the exercise by considering how you will respond to challenges. For example, write out what you would say in the event a client describes a preference you cannot meet (e.g., meeting in a more informal setting, using a treatment approach you are not trained to deliver or you believe to be contraindicated or even harmful). Develop and rehearse several concrete ways for sharing your concerns while simultaneously building and maintaining a collaborative working relationship. As a final step, role-play the responses you develop with colleagues, reflecting on and making adjustments in response to feedback.

Exercise 3: Approaching the Uncomfortable

Principle: 2
Applicability: TDPA Items 4C, E (also applicable to 5Ai, vii, 5Bi)
Purpose
Sometimes therapists struggle with talking about certain topics with their clients. Whether due to apprehension about clients' potential reactions, conflicts with their own personal values or biases, or felt taboos related to certain topics (e.g., money, politics, cultural differences, lack of progress in treatment), the following exercise is designed to provide practice in approaching these uncomfortable areas.

Tasks
As stated in Chapter 1, effective DP relies on "a data-derived identification of 'what' specifically each individual needs to target to improve their performance" (p. 10). While you have already determined a focus on client factors could prove beneficial to improving your results, taking time to gather some

additional information can help in maximizing the effectiveness of exercises related to becoming more skilled in handling uncomfortable conversations. Borrowing from a suggestion in *BR* called the "black box exercise," take a few moments at the end of each workday to reflect on the clients you met. On a sticky note or favorite note-keeping app, write down any instances where you struggled with or avoided certain topics. For the sake of time and efficiency, limit your description to a single instance no longer than a sentence or two of "Twitter length." After a month, review your notes, organizing the collection into themes. Should one recur more often than others, make it the focus of your DP. Alternately, among the themes that emerge, pick one you feel most important or motivated to resolve. Begin with exploring why the topic might be difficult for you. Write down your beliefs and assumptions as well as any concerns you have regarding how clients might interpret you asking about the topic. Next, return to the research review or recommended readings section of the chapter to challenge your beliefs and assumptions and learn new ways of inviting discussions. Set aside time outside the office to script your inquiries and responses, using examples from your daily work. Practice with a colleague. Depending on your comfort level, the partner can provide easy responses or responses that play into your fears about how the client might respond to the question or toward you for asking the question. After 5 minutes of practice, spend another 5 minutes receiving feedback and discussing with your partner how each question sounded.

Exercise 4: Embodiment of a Client

Principle: 3
Applicability: TDPA Item 4E (also applicable to 5Ai, ii, iii, iv, vii, 5Bi)
Purpose
In therapy, as in life, value conflicts and differences between people are inevitable. This exercise is designed to help you recognize, understand, and develop more effective strategies for honoring your clients' values and opinions in session.

Tasks
While writing out your progress notes at the end of the day, recall any client with whom you experienced an explicit or implicit value conflict (e.g., politics, religion, motivation, treatment goal). Close your eyes and picture them in your mind. State *your* view of the conflict out loud, including your thoughts and feelings, as well as why you believe the matter is bothering you so much. Describe in as much detail as possible how the two of you are different from one another. Next, rate your level of frustration with the individual (0 = *no frustration*, 10 = *extreme frustration*).

Eyes open and paper or note-keeping app in hand, write down how your client would describe the conflict. List the experiences or life circumstances that might have led to their beliefs and values. Note how the client might feel about having a conflict in this area with you (their therapist). Consider whether and how, despite any differences, specifically your and your client's goals for meeting are similar. If you struggle to articulate why they believe what they do or how your goals are similar, write out two or three specific ways you will make inquiries at the next visit. Finish by re-rating your level of frustration with the client.

The entire process should take no more than 10 to 15 minutes. Revisit the exercise over several days until a decrease in your frustration is observed. At that point, make a plan for how you are going to approach this conflict in the future with your clients. How will the topic be broached? How will you express empathy and convey understanding?

Exercise 5: Allowing for Differences

Principle: 3
Applicability: TDPA Items 4C, E (also applicable to 5Ai, ii, iv, viii, 5Bi)
Purpose
The purpose of this exercise is to help therapists become more open to the experiences of their clients. It will also aid in expressing empathy and understanding when conflicts occur in sessions. To complete it, you will need to have access to audio or video recordings of your work.

Tasks
As part of your initial assessment and documentation, begin including a formal request to record. Samples of informed consent documents are widely available on the internet. Check to ensure whatever document you adopt meets local and professional regulations regarding recording psychotherapy sessions. No fancy equipment is required. If you have a mobile phone, you have access to a high-quality recording device. Make recording your work the default for all sessions.

At the end of the day, reflect on your meetings with clients, identifying any times when you experienced a conflict, whether openly or internally. Examples might be the reaction you had when a client informed you they had not completed nor could remember the homework assignment, provided you with negative feedback, expressed anger toward you, or shared what you consider a derogatory belief (e.g., homophobic, racist, unnecessarily or inaccurately critical of others or you). Save such recordings and delete the others. Keep a log identifying the type of conflicts reflected in the recordings. Sort for patterns, identifying the most frequent or bothersome.

Next, isolate the section on each recording during which the conflict comes up. Listen and relisten, working purposefully to let go of any judgmental thoughts and feelings. Once done, test your progress by moving on to the next recording and repeating. As a final step, return to the first recording, considering how you responded in the moment. Stop the playback, first reflecting on and then writing out two responses aimed at communicating understanding and empathy.

Exercise 6: Soliciting Feedback

Principle: 4
Applicability: TDPA Items 4B, C, F (also applicable to 5Aviii)
Purpose
Improve your comfort with and ability to solicit feedback from clients.

Tasks
Any of the client factors reviewed in the research section of this chapter may be implicated in clients experiencing low levels of engagement or not making progress in treatment, including (a) treatment preferences or expectations not being met; (b) a lack of understanding of the treatment being provided; (c) a mismatch between the therapy and the client's relational style, identity, values, or beliefs; (d) paucity of social support outside of psychotherapy; and (e) a failure to recognize and reinforce changes in the client's well-being that may not be directly related to work or objectives in therapy. While some of these may reflect a recurring pattern of mistakes on the part of the therapist, many, as pointed out in *BR*, are random. "Psychotherapy," Miller et al. (2020) pointed out, "is cognitively demanding. Any given hour will, therefore, contain myriad (a) 'coulda, woulda, shouldas' as well as (b) an untold number of in-the-moment adjustments" (pp. 104–105). In such instances, improving engagement and outcome depends on increasing therapist responsiveness— doing the right thing at the right moment together with the client. Soliciting feedback via the routine administration of standardized measures has proven particularly helpful in this regard.

As a first step, retrieve the blueprint you created for how you do therapy (described on p. 29 of *BR* and updated on pp. 18–20 in Chapter 1 of this volume). If standardized measures are not included, add them to your map. If you have not developed a script explaining how and why you are using such scales, do so now. At the end of each day, reflect on how you discussed the scores, noting any specific instances where you struggled to communicate clearly or were tempted to forgo discussing the results (e.g., low alliance scores, lack of progress or deterioration, running out of time). Pick one and imagine how you could have addressed client feedback in the moment, committing at least two alternative responses to paper.

Exercise 7: Getting Comfortable With Negative Feedback

Principle: 4
Applicability: TDPA Item 4F (also applicable to 5Ai, ii, iii, iv)
Purpose
For some therapists, receiving critical feedback is difficult. For others, the bigger concern is how to respond most effectively in the moment. This exercise, to be completed with a partner, is designed to increase both comfort and responsiveness to negative client feedback.

Tasks

Take time to reflect on feedback you worry about receiving from clients. It might be broad statements about your overall competence or statements about specific skills or attributes. If you want to make the experience real, first list values and beliefs you have about yourself, your identity, and your work as a clinician (e.g., your effectiveness, skill level, openness, ability to relate to others). Next, ask a trusted colleague to role-play a client who has negative feedback to share based either on one of your specific worries or adopting a perception of you in the feedback that runs counter to how you see yourself. During the process, your job is to listen and reflect, not resolve the feedback expressed by the client, continuing the role-play until *they* feel understood by you. Pay attention to how you feel, repeating the activity at regular intervals until you notice a significant increase in your level of comfort. Should you end up feeling stuck or uncertain about what to do, consult the relevant sections in the research review and additional resources sections of this chapter.

FURTHER READINGS AND RESOURCES

This chapter reviewed available research, identified evidence-based principles, and suggested DP exercises for working with client factors in psychotherapy. Additional research and recommendations can be found in the following:

- Clinical implications and practice suggestions based on the research evidence regarding client factors can be found in Constantino, M. J., Boswell, J. F., & Coyne, A. E. (2021). Patient, therapist, and relational factors. In M. Barkham, W. Lutz, & L. G. Castonguay (Eds.), *Bergin and Garfield's handbook of psychotherapy and behavior change* (7th ed., pp. 229–266). Wiley.

- A thorough review of practice recommendations specific to each of the reviewed client factors along with case examples can be found in Norcross, J. C., & Wampold, B. E. (Eds.). (2019). *Psychotherapy relationships that work: Volume 2. Evidence-based therapist responsiveness* (3rd ed.). Oxford University Press.

- An excellent guide for tailoring psychotherapy to the individual client is Cooper, M., & McLeod, J. (2011). *Pluralistic counselling and psychotherapy.* SAGE.

- A recently published resource for accommodating client preferences is Norcross, J. C., & Cooper, M. (2021). *Personalizing psychotherapy: Assessing and accommodating patient preferences.* American Psychological Association.

- A discussion of using these principles to encourage psychotherapy engagement along with case examples can be found in Swift, J. K., & Greenberg, R. P. (2015). *Premature termination in psychotherapy: Strategies for engaging clients and improving outcomes.* American Psychological Association.

- Specific evidence-based strategies for using client strengths and resources, including chance-change producing events and pretreatment change, can be found in Miller, S., Duncan, B., & Hubble, M. (1995). *Escape from Babel: Toward a unifying language for psychotherapy practice.* Norton.

- Detailed instructions for incorporating routine outcome measurement into clinical work is available in Prescott, D., Maeschalck, C., & Miller, S. (Eds.). (2017). *Feedback-informed treatment in clinical practice: Reaching for excellence.* American Psychological Association.

REFERENCES

American Psychological Association Presidential Task Force on Evidence-Based Practice. (2006). Evidence-based practice in psychology. *American Psychologist, 61*(4), 271–285. https://doi.org/10.1037/0003-066X.61.4.271

Arnkoff, D. B., Glass, C. R., & Shapiro, S. J. (2002). Expectations and preferences. In J. C. Norcross (Ed.), *Psychotherapy relationships that work* (pp. 335–356). Oxford University Press.

Atchley, P. (2010, December 21). You can't multitask, so stop trying. *Harvard Business Review.* www.hbr.org/2010/12/you-cant-multi-task-so-stop-tr

Beutler, L. E., Edwards, C., & Someah, K. (2018). Adapting psychotherapy to patient reactance level: A meta-analytic review. *Journal of Clinical Psychology, 74*(11), 1952–1963. https://doi.org/10.1002/jclp.22682

Bohart, A. C., & Wade, A. G. (2013). The client in psychotherapy. In M. J. Lambert (Ed.), *Bergin and Garfield's handbook of psychotherapy and behavior change* (6th ed., pp. 219–257). Wiley.

Brehm, S. S., & Brehm, J. W. (1981). *Psychological reactance: A theory of freedom and control.* Academic Press.

Budge, S. L., & Moradi, B. (2018). Attending to gender in psychotherapy: Understanding and incorporating systems of power. *Journal of Clinical Psychology, 74*(11), 2014–2027. https://doi.org/10.1002/jclp.22686

Cabral, R. R., & Smith, T. B. (2011). Racial/ethnic matching of clients and therapists in mental health services: A meta-analytic review of preferences, perceptions, and outcomes. *Journal of Counseling Psychology, 58*(4), 537–554. https://doi.org/10.1037/a0025266

Captari, L. E., Hook, J. N., Hoyt, W., Davis, D. E., McElroy-Heltzel, S. E., & Worthington, E. L., Jr. (2018). Integrating clients' religion and spirituality within psychotherapy: A comprehensive meta-analysis. *Journal of Clinical Psychology, 74*(11), 1938–1951. https://doi.org/10.1002/jclp.22681

Chambless, D. L., & Hollon, S. D. (1998). Defining empirically supported therapies. *Journal of Consulting and Clinical Psychology, 66*(1), 7–18. https://doi.org/10.1037/0022-006X.66.1.7

Chow, D. (2022, February 28). Take note of these 4 perennial factors of your clients. *Frontiers of Psychotherapist Development.* https://darylchow.com/frontiers/4s/

Chow, D., & Miller, S. D. (2022). *Taxonomy of Deliberate Practice Activities in Psychotherapy—Therapist Version* (Version 6). International Center for Clinical Excellence.

Constantine, M. G. (2007). Racial microaggressions against African American clients in cross-racial counseling relationships. *Journal of Counseling Psychology, 54*(1), 1–16. https://doi.org/10.1037/0022-0167.54.1.1

Constantino, M. J., Boswell, J. F., & Coyne, A. E. (2021). Patient, therapist, and relational factors. In M. Barkham, W. Lutz, & L. G. Castonguay (Eds.), *Bergin and Garfield's handbook of psychotherapy and behavior change* (7th ed., pp. 229–266). Wiley.

Costantino, G., Malgady, R. G., & Rogler, L. H. (1986). Cuento therapy: A culturally sensitive modality for Puerto Rican children. *Journal of Consulting and Clinical Psychology*, *54*(5), 639–645. https://doi.org/10.1037/0022-006X.54.5.639

Cooper, M., & McLeod, J. (2011). *Pluralistic counselling and psychotherapy*. SAGE.

Cross, W. E., Jr. (2021). *Black identity viewed from a barber's chair*. Temple University Press.

Davis, D. E., DeBlaere, C., Owen, J., Hook, J. N., Rivera, D. P., Choe, E., Van Tongeren, D. R., Worthington, E. L., Jr., & Placeres, V. (2018). The multicultural orientation framework: A narrative review. *Psychotherapy*, *55*(1), 89–100. https://doi.org/10.1037/pst0000160

Dimmick, A., Trusty, W., & Swift, J. K. (2021). Client preferences for religious/spiritual integration and matching in psychotherapy. *Spirituality in Clinical Practice*. Advance online publication. https://doi.org/10.1037/scp0000269

Dour, H. J., Chorpita, B. F., Lee, S., Weisz, J. R., & the Research Network on Youth Mental Health. (2013). Sudden gains as a long-term predictor of treatment improvement among children in community mental health organizations. *Behaviour Research and Therapy*, *51*(9), 564–572. https://doi.org/10.1016/j.brat.2013.05.012

Drinane, J. M., Owen, J., & Kopta, S. M. (2016). Racial/ethnic disparities in psychotherapy: Does the outcome matter? *TPM*, *23*(4), 531–544.

Drinane, J. M., Roberts, T., Winderman, K., Freeman, V. F., & Wang, Y. W. (2022). The myth of the safe space: Sexual orientation disparities in therapist effectiveness. *Journal of Counseling Psychology*. Advance online publication. https://doi.org/10.1037/cou0000584

Duffy, M. E., Henkel, K. E., & Earnshaw, V. A. (2016). Transgender clients' experiences of eating disorder treatment. *Journal of LGBT Issues in Counseling*, *10*(3), 136–149. https://doi.org/10.1080/15538605.2016.1177806

Duncan, B. L., Miller, S. D., Wampold, B. E., & Hubble, M. A. (Eds.). (2010). *The heart and soul of change: Delivering what works in therapy* (2nd ed.). American Psychological Association. https://doi.org/10.1037/12075-000

Elder, A. B. (2016). Experiences of older transgender and gender nonconforming adults in psychotherapy: A qualitative study. *Psychology of Sexual Orientation and Gender Diversity*, *3*(2), 180–186. https://doi.org/10.1037/sgd0000154

Fancher, R. T. (1995). *Cultures of healing: Correcting the image of American mental health care*. W. H. Freeman/Times Books/Henry Holt.

Flückiger, C., Del Re, A. C., Wampold, B. E., & Horvath, A. O. (2018). The alliance in adult psychotherapy: A meta-analytic synthesis. *Psychotherapy*, *55*(4), 316–340. https://doi.org/10.1037/pst0000172

Garfield, S. L. (1994). Research on client variables in psychotherapy. In A. E. Bergin & S. L. Garfield (Eds.), *Handbook of psychotherapy and behavior change* (4th ed., pp. 190–228). Wiley.

Gassmann, D., & Grawe, K. (2006). General change mechanisms: The relation between problem activation and resource activation in successful and unsuccessful therapeutic interactions. *Clinical Psychology & Psychotherapy*, *13*(1), 1–11. https://doi.org/10.1002/cpp.442

Goldfried, M. R. (1980). Toward the delineation of therapeutic change principles. *American Psychologist*, *35*(11), 991–999. https://doi.org/10.1037/0003-066X.35.11.991

Hayes, J. A., McAleavey, A. A., Castonguay, L. G., & Locke, B. D. (2016). Psychotherapists' outcomes with White and racial/ethnic minority clients: First, the good news. *Journal of Counseling Psychology*, *63*(3), 261–268. https://doi.org/10.1037/cou0000098

Hayes, J. A., Owen, J., & Bieschke, K. J. (2015). Therapist differences in symptom change with racial/ethnic minority clients. *Psychotherapy*, *52*(3), 308–314. https://doi.org/10.1037/a0037957

Hook, J. N., Davis, D., Owen, J., & DeBlaere, C. (2017). *Cultural humility: Engaging diverse identities in therapy*. American Psychological Association. https://doi.org/10.1037/0000037-000

Hook, J. N., Davis, D. E., Owen, J., Worthington, E. L., Jr., & Utsey, S. O. (2013). Cultural humility: Measuring openness to culturally diverse clients. *Journal of Counseling Psychology, 60*(3), 353–366. https://doi.org/10.1037/a0032595

Hook, J. N., Farrell, J. E., Davis, D. E., DeBlaere, C., Van Tongeren, D. R., & Utsey, S. O. (2016). Cultural humility and racial microaggressions in counseling. *Journal of Counseling Psychology, 63*(3), 269–277. https://doi.org/10.1037/cou0000114

Horvath, A. O., Del Re, A. C., Flückiger, C., & Symonds, D. (2011). Alliance in individual psychotherapy. *Psychotherapy, 48*(1), 9–16. https://doi.org/10.1037/a0022186

Howard, K. I., Kopta, S. M., Krause, M. S., & Orlinsky, D. E. (1986). The dose–effect relationship in psychotherapy. *American Psychologist, 41*(2), 159–164. https://doi.org/10.1037/0003-066X.41.2.159

Hubble, M. A., Duncan, B. L., & Miller, S. D. (Eds.). (1999). *The heart and soul of change: What works in therapy.* American Psychological Association. https://doi.org/10.1037/11132-000

Huey, S. J., Jr., Tilley, J. L., Jones, E. O., & Smith, C. A. (2014). The contribution of cultural competence to evidence-based care for ethnically diverse populations. *Annual Review of Clinical Psychology, 10*(1), 305–338. https://doi.org/10.1146/annurev-clinpsy-032813-153729

Ibrahim, N., Michail, M., & Callaghan, P. (2014). The strengths based approach as a service delivery model for severe mental illness: A meta-analysis of clinical trials. *BMC Psychiatry, 14*(1), 243. https://doi.org/10.1186/s12888-014-0243-6

Imel, Z. E., Baldwin, S., Atkins, D. C., Owen, J., Baardseth, T., & Wampold, B. E. (2011). Racial/ethnic disparities in therapist effectiveness: A conceptualization and initial study of cultural competence. *Journal of Counseling Psychology, 58*(3), 290–298. https://doi.org/10.1037/a0023284

Krebs, P., Norcross, J. C., Nicholson, J. M., & Prochaska, J. O. (2018). Stages of change and psychotherapy outcomes: A review and meta-analysis. *Journal of Clinical Psychology, 74*(11), 1964–1979. https://doi.org/10.1002/jclp.22683

Larrison, C. R., Schoppelrey, S. L., Hack-Ritzo, S., & Korr, W. S. (2011). Clinician factors related to outcome differences between black and white patients at CMHCs. *Psychiatric Services, 62*(5), 525–531. https://doi.org/10.1176/ps.62.5.pss6205_0525

Lawson, D. (1994). Identifying pretreatment change. *Journal of Counseling and Development, 72*(3), 244–248. https://doi.org/10.1002/j.1556-6676.1994.tb00929.x

Leibert, T. W., Smith, J. B., & Agaskar, V. R. (2011). Relationship between the working alliance and social support on counseling outcome. *Journal of Clinical Psychology, 67*(7), 709–719. https://doi.org/10.1002/jclp.20800

Levy, K. N., Kivity, Y., Johnson, B. N., & Gooch, C. V. (2018). Adult attachment as a predictor and moderator of psychotherapy outcome: A meta-analysis. *Journal of Clinical Psychology, 74*(11), 1996–2013. https://doi.org/10.1002/jclp.22685

Longabaugh, R., Wirtz, P. W., Zweben, A., & Stout, R. L. (1998). Network support for drinking, Alcoholics Anonymous and long-term matching effects. *Addiction, 93*(9), 1313–1333. https://doi.org/10.1046/j.1360-0443.1998.93913133.x

Malins, S., Moghaddam, N., Morriss, R., Schröder, T., Brown, P., & Boycott, N. (2021). Predicting outcomes and sudden gains from initial in-session interactions during remote cognitive-behavioural therapy for severe health anxiety. *Clinical Psychology & Psychotherapy, 28*(4), 891–906. https://doi.org/10.1002/cpp.2543

Martinez, J. S., Smith, T. B., & Barlow, S. H. (2007). Spiritual interventions in psychotherapy: Evaluations by highly religious clients. *Journal of Clinical Psychology, 63*(10), 943–960. https://doi.org/10.1002/jclp.20399

McHugh, R. K., Whitton, S. W., Peckham, A. D., Welge, J. A., & Otto, M. W. (2013). Patient preference for psychological vs pharmacologic treatment of psychiatric disorders: A meta-analytic review. *The Journal of Clinical Psychiatry, 74*(6), 595–602. https://doi.org/10.4088/JCP.12r07757

Miller, C. H., Lane, L. T., Deatrick, L. M., Young, A. M., & Potts, K. A. (2007). Psychological reactance and promotional health messages: The effects of controlling language, lexical concreteness, and the restoration of freedom. *Human Communication Research, 33*(2), 219–240. https://doi.org/10.1111/j.1468-2958.2007.00297.x

Miller, S., Duncan, B., & Hubble, M. (1995). *Escape from Babel: Toward a unifying language for psychotherapy practice.* Norton.

Miller, S. D., & Hubble, M. A. (2017). How psychotherapy lost its magick: The art of healing in an age of science. *Psychotherapy Networker, 41*(2), 28–37, 60–61.

Miller, S. D., Hubble, M. A., & Chow, D. (2020). *Better results: Using deliberate practice to improve therapeutic effectiveness.* American Psychological Association. https://doi.org/10.1037/0000191-000

Monks, G. M. (1996). A meta-analysis of role induction studies. *Dissertation Abstracts International: Section B. The Sciences and Engineering, 56*(12-B), 7051.

Moradi, B., & Budge, S. L. (2018). Engaging in LGBQ+ affirmative psychotherapies with all clients: Defining themes and practices. *Journal of Clinical Psychology, 74*(11), 2028–2042. https://doi.org/10.1002/jclp.22687

Norcross, J. C., & Cooper, M. (2021). *Personalizing psychotherapy: Assessing and accommodating patient preferences.* American Psychological Association. https://doi.org/10.1037/0000221-000

Norcross, J. C., Krebs, P. M., & Prochaska, J. O. (2011). Stages of change. In J. C. Norcross (Ed.), *Psychotherapy relationships that work* (2nd ed., pp. 279–300). Oxford University Press. https://doi.org/10.1093/acprof:oso/9780199737208.003.0014

Norcross, J. C., & Wampold, B. E. (2018). A new therapy for each patient: Evidence-based relationships and responsiveness. *Journal of Clinical Psychology, 74*(11), 1889–1906. https://doi.org/10.1002/jclp.22678

Norcross, J. C., & Wampold, B. E. (Eds.). (2019). *Psychotherapy relationships that work: Volume 2. Evidence-based therapist responsiveness* (3rd ed.). Oxford University Press.

Oldham, M., Kellett, S., Miles, E., & Sheeran, P. (2012). Interventions to increase attendance at psychotherapy: A meta-analysis of randomized controlled trials. *Journal of Consulting and Clinical Psychology, 80*(5), 928–939. https://doi.org/10.1037/a0029630

Owen, J. (2013). Early career perspectives on psychotherapy research and practice: Psychotherapist effects, multicultural orientation, and couple interventions. *Psychotherapy, 50*(4), 496–502. https://doi.org/10.1037/a0034617

Owen, J., Drinane, J., Tao, K. W., Adelson, J. L., Hook, J. N., Davis, D., & Fookune, N. (2017). Racial/ethnic disparities in client unilateral termination: The role of therapists' cultural comfort. *Psychotherapy Research, 27*(1), 102–111. https://doi.org/10.1080/10503307.2015.1078517

Owen, J., Imel, Z., Adelson, J., & Rodolfa, E. (2012). 'No-show': Therapist racial/ethnic disparities in client unilateral termination. *Journal of Counseling Psychology, 59*(2), 314–320. https://doi.org/10.1037/a0027091

Owen, J., Imel, Z., Tao, K. W., Wampold, B., Smith, A., & Rodolfa, E. (2011). Cultural ruptures in short-term therapy: Working alliance as a mediator between clients' perceptions of microaggressions and therapy outcomes. *Counselling & Psychotherapy Research, 11*(3), 204–212. https://doi.org/10.1080/14733145.2010.491551

Owen, J., Jordan, T., Turner, D., Davis, D., Hook, J., & Leach, M. (2014). Therapists' multicultural orientation: Cultural humility, spiritual/religious identity, and therapy outcomes. *Journal of Psychology and Theology, 42*(1), 91–98. https://doi.org/10.1177/009164711404200110

Owen, J., Tao, K., Drinane, J., Hook, J., Davis, D., & Foo Kune, N. (2016). Client perceptions of therapists' multicultural orientation: Cultural (missed) opportunities and cultural humility. *Professional Psychology, Research and Practice, 47*(1), 30–37. https://doi.org/10.1037/pro0000046

Owen, J., Tao, K., & Rodolfa, E. (2010). Microaggressions and women in short-term psychotherapy: Initial evidence. *The Counseling Psychologist, 38*(7), 923–946. https://doi.org/10.1177/0011000010376093

Owen, J., Wong, Y. J., & Rodolfa, E. (2009). Empirical search for psychotherapists' gender competence in psychotherapy. *Psychotherapy, 46*(4), 448–458. https://doi.org/10.1037/a0017958

Prescott, D., Maeschalck, C., & Miller, S. (Eds.). (2017). *Feedback-informed treatment in clinical practice: Reaching for excellence.* American Psychological Association. https://doi.org/10.1037/0000039-000

Prochaska, J. O., & DiClemente, C. C. (1983). Stages and processes of self-change of smoking: Toward an integrative model of change. *Journal of Consulting and Clinical Psychology, 51*(3), 390–395. https://doi.org/10.1037/0022-006X.51.3.390

Project MATCH. (1997). Matching alcoholism treatments to client heterogeneity: Project MATCH posttreatment drinking outcomes. *Journal of Studies on Alcohol, 58*(1), 7–29. https://doi.org/10.15288/jsa.1997.58.7

Reuterlov, H., Lofgren, T., Nordstrom, K., Ternstrom, A., & Miller, S. D. (2000). What is better? A preliminary investigation of between-session change. *Journal of Systemic Therapies, 19*(1), 111–115. https://doi.org/10.1521/jsyt.2000.19.1.111

Reyes-Rodríguez, M. L., Baucom, D. H., & Bulik, C. M. (2014). Culturally sensitive intervention for Latina women with eating disorders: A case study. *Revista Mexicana de Trastornos Alimentarios, 5*(2), 136–146. https://doi.org/10.1016/S2007-1523(14)72009-9

Roehrle, B., & Strouse, J. (2008). Influence of social support on success of therapeutic interventions: A meta-analytic review. *Psychotherapy, 45*(4), 464–476. https://doi.org/10.1037/a0014333

Rose, E. M., Westefeld, J. S., & Ansely, T. N. (2001). Spiritual issues in counseling: Clients' beliefs and preferences. *Journal of Counseling Psychology, 48*(1), 61–71. https://doi.org/10.1037/0022-0167.48.1.61

Rosmarin, D. H., Forester, B. P., Shassian, D. M., Webb, C. A., & Björgvinsson, T. (2015). Interest in spiritually integrated psychotherapy among acute psychiatric patients. *Journal of Consulting and Clinical Psychology, 83*(6), 1149–1153. https://doi.org/10.1037/ccp0000046

Shalom, J. G., & Aderka, I. M. (2020). A meta-analysis of sudden gains in psychotherapy: Outcome and moderators. *Clinical Psychology Review.* Advance online publication. https://doi.org/10.1016/j.cpr.2020.101827

Shelton, K., & Delgado-Romero, E. A. (2013). Sexual orientation microaggressions: The experience of lesbian, gay, bisexual, and queer clients in psychotherapy. *Psychology of Sexual Orientation and Gender Diversity, 1*(S), 59–70.

Soto, A., Smith, T. B., Griner, D., Domenech Rodríguez, M., & Bernal, G. (2018). Cultural adaptations and therapist multicultural competence: Two meta-analytic reviews. *Journal of Clinical Psychology, 74*(11), 1907–1923. https://doi.org/10.1002/jclp.22679

Stiles, W. B., & Horvath, A. O. (2017). Appropriate responsiveness as a contribution to therapist effects. In L. G. Castonguay & C. E. Hill (Eds.), *How and why are some therapists better than others? Understanding therapist effects* (pp. 71–84). American Psychological Association. https://doi.org/10.1037/0000034-005

Stiles, W. B., Leach, C., Barkham, M., Lucock, M., Iveson, S., Shapiro, D. A., Iveson, M., & Hardy, G. E. (2003). Early sudden gains in psychotherapy under routine clinic conditions: Practice-based evidence. *Journal of Consulting and Clinical Psychology, 71*(1), 14–21. https://doi.org/10.1037/0022-006X.71.1.14

Sue, D. W., Arredondo, P., & McDavis, R. J. (1992). Multicultural counseling competencies and standards: A call to the profession. *Journal of Counseling and Development, 70*(4), 477–486. https://doi.org/10.1002/j.1556-6676.1992.tb01642.x

Sue, S. (2006). Cultural competency: From philosophy to research and practice. *Journal of Community Psychology, 34*(2), 237–245. https://doi.org/10.1002/jcop.20095

Swift, J. K., & Callahan, J. L. (2008). A delay-discounting measure of great expectations and the effectiveness of psychotherapy. *Professional Psychology, Research and Practice, 39*(6), 581–588. https://doi.org/10.1037/0735-7028.39.6.581

Swift, J. K., & Callahan, J. L. (2010). A comparison of client preferences for intervention empirical support versus common therapy variables. *Journal of Clinical Psychology, 66*(12), 1217–1231. https://doi.org/10.1002/jclp.20720

Swift, J. K., & Callahan, J. L. (2011). Decreasing treatment dropout by addressing expectations for treatment length. *Psychotherapy Research, 21*(2), 193–200. https://doi.org/10.1080/10503307.2010.541294

Swift, J. K., Callahan, J. L., Cooper, M., & Parkin, S. R. (2018). The impact of accommodating client preference in psychotherapy: A meta-analysis. *Journal of Clinical Psychology, 74*(11), 1924–1937. https://doi.org/10.1002/jclp.22680

Swift, J. K., Callahan, J. L., Tompkins, K. A., Connor, D. R., & Dunn, R. (2015). A delay-discounting measure of preference for racial/ethnic matching in psychotherapy. *Psychotherapy, 52*(3), 315–320. https://doi.org/10.1037/pst0000019

Swift, J. K., & Greenberg, R. P. (2015). *Premature termination in psychotherapy: Strategies for engaging clients and improving outcomes.* American Psychological Association. https://doi.org/10.1037/14469-000

Swift, J. K., Mullins, R. H., Penix, E. A., Roth, K. L., & Trusty, W. T. (2021). The importance of listening to patient preferences when making mental health care decisions. *World Psychiatry, 20*(3), 316–317. https://doi.org/10.1002/wps.20912

Tang, T. Z., & DeRubeis, R. J. (1999). Sudden gains and critical sessions in cognitive-behavioral therapy for depression. *Journal of Consulting and Clinical Psychology, 67*(6), 894–904. https://doi.org/10.1037/0022-006X.67.6.894

Tao, K. W., Whiteley, A., Noel, N., & Ozawa-Kirk, J. (2016, August 4–7). White therapy dyads and missed cultural opportunities. In S. M. Hoover (Chair), *Social justice in counseling—opportunities to consider intersectionality and invisible difference* [Symposium]. American Psychological Association 124th Annual Convention, Denver, CO, United States.

Tompkins, K. A., Swift, J. K., Rousmaniere, T. G., & Whipple, J. L. (2017). The relationship between clients' depression etiological beliefs and psychotherapy orientation preferences, expectations, and credibility beliefs. *Psychotherapy, 54*(2), 201–206. https://doi.org/10.1037/pst0000070

Trusty, W. T., Swift, J. K., Winkeljohn Black, S., Dimmick, A. A., & Penix, E. A. (2022). Religious microaggressions in psychotherapy: A mixed methods examination of client perspectives. *Psychotherapy.* Advance online publication. https://doi.org/10.1037/pst0000408

Wampold, B. E., & Imel, Z. E. (2015). *The great psychotherapy debate: The evidence for what makes psychotherapy work* (2nd ed.). Routledge/Taylor & Francis Group.

Weiner-Davis, M., de Shazer, S., & Gingerich, W. (1987). Building on pretreatment change to construct the therapeutic solution. *Journal of Marital and Family Therapy, 13*(4), 359–363. https://doi.org/10.1111/j.1752-0606.1987.tb00717.x

Windle, E., Tee, H., Sabitova, A., Jovanovic, N., Priebe, S., & Carr, C. (2020). Association of patient treatment preference with dropout and clinical outcomes in adult psychosocial mental health interventions: A systematic review and meta-analysis. *JAMA Psychiatry, 77*(3), 294–302. https://doi.org/10.1001/jamapsychiatry.2019.3750

Therapist Factors

Helene A. Nissen-Lie, Erkki Heinonen, and Jaime Delgadillo

The essence of therapy is embodied in the therapist.

—BRUCE E. WAMPOLD AND ZAC E. IMEL,
THE GREAT PSYCHOTHERAPY DEBATE

DECISION POINT

Begin here if you have read the book *Better Results* (*BR*) and

- are routinely measuring your performance *and*
- have collected sufficient data to establish a reliable, evidence-based profile of your therapeutic effectiveness *and*
- have completed the Taxonomy of Deliberate Practice Activities in Psychotherapy *and*
- need help developing deliberate practice exercises that leverage the therapist's contribution to outcome.

To understand the effectiveness of treatment, mainstream psychotherapy researchers have traditionally focused on investigating techniques or strategies associated with specific schools of therapy (psychodynamic, cognitive behavioral, and humanistic), often matched to client factors (e.g., diagnoses) at the expense of understanding the impact of the provider of the treatment, namely, the therapist (see Barkham & Lambert, 2021).

https://doi.org/10.1037/0000358-005
The Field Guide to Better Results: Evidence-Based Exercises to Improve Therapeutic Effectiveness,
S. D. Miller, D. Chow, S. Malins, and M. A. Hubble (Editors)

Over the years, many leading theorists have pointed to the crucial role therapists play in the outcome of care. As early as the 1930s, Saul Rosenzweig (1936) said,

> It may be said that given a therapist who has an effective personality and who consistently adheres in his treatment to a system of concepts which he has mastered and which is in one significant way or another adapted to the problems of the sick personality, then it is of comparatively little consequence what particular method that therapist uses. (pp. 414–415)

In the late 1950s, another pioneer in the field, Carl Rogers (1957), proposed that the positive effects of psychotherapy would crucially depend on the ability of the therapist to meet their clients with empathy, unconditional positive regard, and genuineness (i.e., congruence). In the 1960s, Jerome Frank proposed a common factors model that emphasized the therapeutic alliance, the fostering of hope, and the specific influence of the healer's persuasiveness as crucial factors that promote change (Frank, 1961; Frank & Frank, 1991).

While theoretical accounts of how clinicians influence the processes and outcomes of therapy date back to the first half of the last century, it is only in the last 30 years that researchers have explicitly focused on therapist effects and their determinants (e.g., Baldwin & Imel, 2013; Barkham et al., 2017; Crits-Christoph et al., 1991; Wampold & Owen, 2021).

One reason it took so much time to recognize the impact individual therapists have on the effectiveness of treatment was the influence of the medical model. Specific therapeutic interventions were seen as responsible for therapeutic results. In *The Great Psychotherapy Debate*, Bruce Wampold (2001) questioned the empirical support for thinking of psychological approaches as analogs of medical treatments (see also Wampold & Imel, 2015). "On the contrary," he argued, "the scientific evidence overwhelmingly supports a model of psychotherapy that gives primacy to the healing context" (p. xii). While acknowledging therapist effects do not negate the importance of specific interventions, psychotherapy, evidence shows, cannot be likened to drugs that work independently of the provider (or the recipient, for that matter). Rather, success depends on the therapist creating and maintaining engagement in processes that often require significant effort on the part of the client: that of changing habitual but dysfunctional ways of coping with life events, both past and present.

The contextual understanding Wampold (2001) proposed included a growing number of demonstrably effective factors relevant across different models of psychotherapy, which are included in the Taxonomy of Deliberate Practice Activities in Psychotherapy (TDPA; Chow & Miller, 2022; see Appendix A, this volume)—the tool that informs the organization of this book. These empirically supported domains include structure, hope, and expectancy; the therapeutic relationship; client factors; and therapist factors. This chapter focuses on the last of these factors, first reviewing studies documenting the therapist skills, characteristics, and qualities associated with positive outcomes and then distilling the research findings into a series of evidence-based principles. Consistent with other chapters, the findings and principles are operationalized in a series of practical exercises clinicians can apply in their deliberate practice (DP) efforts (Miller, Hubble, & Chow, 2020). Focusing on the therapist can, it must be recognized, give rise to uncertainty and anxiety: Do I have what it takes? Before proceeding, it might be comforting to know the findings point more to an *approach* to practice, personal development, and clinical work rather than a set of well-defined and stable *traits*.

REVIEW OF THE RESEARCH

Today, it is regarded as well-established that individual therapists account for a significant proportion of client outcomes in psychotherapy. Referred to as *therapist effects* (Baldwin & Imel, 2013; Wampold & Owen, 2021), meta-analytic reviews show, in both randomized controlled trials and naturalistic studies, around 5% of the variance in client outcomes is attributable to differences between practitioners (Baldwin & Imel, 2013; Johns et al., 2019; Wampold & Owen, 2021). Just how important is the clinician? Given that treatment, in total, explains about 14% of the difference in outcome between clients, the contribution made by the individual therapists can only be thought of as critical (Baldwin & Imel, 2013)—accounting for about one third of the total variability in effect.

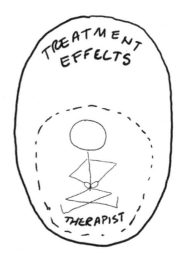

A few key studies can be used to demonstrate the importance of the therapist. Okiishi et al. (2003), for example, found recovery rates of the most effective therapists were twice those attained by the least helpful. Meanwhile, analyses of routine practice data conducted by Saxon and Barkham (2012) showed that 15% more clients recovered when seen by an "average" rather than the least effective clinicians in their sample. The authors further showed the variability in outcomes due to therapists was greater when clients' pretreatment clinical symptoms were more severe, indicating "who" provides treatment is a critical consideration with more severe cases. Similar findings were reported by Firth et al. (2015), whose research showed the more effective practitioners (i.e., above average) achieved almost double the amount of change per session compared with their "below average" counterparts. Here again, the difference in outcomes between therapists was especially pronounced with the more functionally impaired.

What can practitioners learn from such findings about achieving better results? One key quality of the most effective therapists, it appears, is *consistency*. Some studies have shown that therapists are consistent across outcome domains

(Nissen-Lie et al., 2016), while other studies have demonstrated therapists are not equally effective across client-presenting problems (e.g., Kraus et al., 2011) or populations (e.g., racial or ethnic minorities; Hayes et al., 2016; Imel et al., 2011; Owen et al., 2015). Similar inconsistencies were reported in a recent trial by Constantino, Boswell, Coyne, et al. (2021), which also found that therapist self-ratings were unrelated to their actual effectiveness with various client subgroups and that clients did no better when they were seen by therapists who perceived themselves as skilled in helping people with particular presenting concerns.

After finding that clinicians who achieved similar results *across* clients were also *more* effective, Owen and colleagues (2019) concluded any definition of psychotherapeutic expertise needed to include consistency over time *and* within caseload. Their study is notable for its large and diverse sample size, nearly 38,000 clients and over 800 therapists (see also Delgadillo et al., 2020; Nissen-Lie et al., 2016; Wampold & Brown, 2005). Taken together with new research documenting the existence of meaningful differences between therapists in their client's magnitude and rate of change *early* in therapists' careers, the evidence highlights the need for and potential utility of DP at the beginning of professional training (Edmondstone et al., 2022).

In sum, numerous studies applying appropriate statistical methods (e.g., multilevel modeling) to large samples have established that therapists do differ in their clinical effectiveness—to a degree that makes a substantial difference in the lives of clients and the overall effectiveness of mental health services. Hence, the most effective therapists are consistently effective over time, across outcome domains, and across clients with diverse clinical and demographic

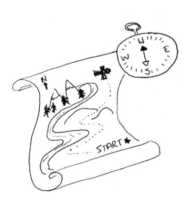

FIELD GUIDE TIP

Professional musicians work at achieving consistency in their performance using a simple tool: a matchbox. While practicing, each time they get the timing or technical aspects of a particular stanza, chord, or progression correct, one match is removed from the box. If an error is made along the way, all the matches are returned, and the process starts over. Practice of the targeted aspect of the music is ended when the matchbox is empty.

Consider how you might adapt or integrate the "matchbox" method in your deliberate practice.

characteristics. By contrast, the majority (around 70%) of practitioners are not significantly different from average, and their effectiveness across time, problem types, and client groups is less stable.

The critical question is what findings about differences between therapists means for training, supervision, and professional development. Like all people, clinicians have some stable characteristics that are trait-like and shaped over the life course. Others are state-like, more situational, and modifiable. Unfortunately, at present, little research exists on whether or how such therapist dispositions might be changed through focused and intensive training or, for example, engagement in personal therapy—although a small number of studies show both avenues to be promising (e.g., Anderson et al., 2016; Orlinsky & Rønnestad, 2005; Ziede & Norcross, 2020).

Potentially relevant attributes may be related to clinicians' lives outside of therapy (i.e., attitudes, values, personality, interpersonal skills). Indeed, some of these qualities measured before training predict clinical outcomes a year later (see Anderson et al., 2016, and later in this section). Clearly, education and training also shape relational manner and style; perceptual, conceptual, and thinking skills; as well as expertise in carrying out particular techniques and interventions (Knox & Hill, 2021). Curiously, the latter dominates most instructional textbooks and training courses despite "the person of the therapist" being unavoidably intertwined with professional performance. This review continues with both aspects, beginning with therapists' professional characteristics (i.e., those developed specifically for therapy work) and ending with a summary of the personal qualities (i.e., those describing the therapist in their overall life) associated with treatment outcome.

Therapists' Professional Characteristics

Asked what qualifies someone to work as a psychotherapist, the average layperson will likely cite professional training, licensure, and experience. As reviewed in Chapter 1 of this field guide, a career in the field of mental health requires a significant investment of time and money, college and graduate school courses, thousands of hours of supervised practice, and passing a licensing exam, to name but a few. And yet, various studies show professional training and discipline (e.g., psychologist, nurse, social worker, professional counselor, medical doctor) do not explain between-therapist differences in effectiveness. Neither, it appears, do clinical qualifications, licensure, hours of supervision, or specialization (see research reviews in Chapters 1, 5, and 7). Also, as cited by practitioners and clients alike, clinical experience is not a reliable predictor of better results (Beutler et al., 2004). In fact, an empirical study found that therapist effectiveness may deteriorate over time (Goldberg, Rousmaniere, et al., 2016; see Table 4.1 for a summary of the professional qualities that do not make a difference). To this list of professional characteristics with little, no, or mixed empirical support, Wampold and Owen (2021), in a recent, comprehensive review of the literature for the *Handbook of Psychotherapy*

TABLE 4.1. Professional Characteristics and Treatment Outcome

Professional characteristic	Impact on outcome
Discipline	No correlation
Theoretical orientation or integration	No correlation
Licensure or certification	No correlation
Supervision	No correlation
Clinical experience	No correlation
Adherence to treatment manuals	Mixed evidence
Therapist rated specialization or skills	No correlation
Rated competence	Mixed evidence
Consistency in outcome	Predictive
Empathic ability or responsiveness	Predictive
Management of countertransference reactions	Predictive
Facilitative interpersonal skills	Predictive
Engagement in deliberate practice	Promising

and Behavior Change, added theoretical orientation and integration, adherence to treatment manuals, and rated competence (see also Webb et al., 2010), even if some recent work points to the potential effects of therapeutic competence in the delivery of therapeutic techniques on outcomes (Power et al., 2022).

Given the foregoing, what professional characteristics can a therapist focus on and develop to become more effective? One hypothesis is that crude variables such as clinical experience or qualifications are poor proxy indicators of therapeutic skillfulness. Another related possibility is that subtle yet discrete interpersonal and attitudinal attributes may be more important than experience when it comes to helping clients.

With regard to the latter, consider research on therapists' perceptions of their skillfulness (e.g., self-confidence; see Heinonen & Nissen-Lie, 2020). In contrast to what one might hope, multiple studies confirm a tendency among

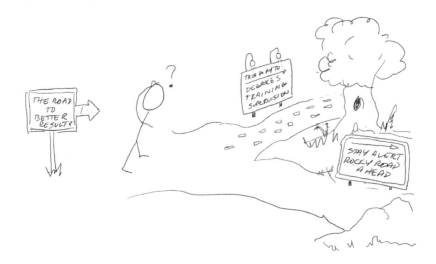

practitioners to overestimate their effectiveness (Chow et al., 2015; Walfish et al., 2012). Ziem and Hoyer (2020) documented the consequences resulting from the disconnect between therapist actual and perceived impact on client functioning and well-being. Comparing therapists' assessments of their clients' progress with clients' measured improvement, they found more modest or conservative therapist estimations (relative to their clients' actual improvement) predicted *larger* reductions of clients' symptoms and greater improvements in quality of life.

At first, such findings appear to provide support for humility as an important characteristic of effective therapists. Research findings on this construct are mixed, however, with some studies reporting that therapists with higher professional self-doubt (i.e., lacking confidence in their ability to be helpful, feeling unsure about the best way to work with a given client) have better alliances and outcomes (Nissen-Lie et al., 2010, 2013), with others showing no association (Delgadillo et al., 2022; Odyniec et al., 2019). A plausible interpretation of these seemingly contradictory findings is that therapist doubt and humility are not, in and of themselves, curative but rather dispositional traits that engender other behaviors leading to greater client engagement and improvement. For example, in two separate studies, Lutz et al. (2015) and de Jong et al. (2012) found positive therapist attitudes toward client feedback regarding the process and effectiveness of care predicted better outcomes. Clearly, a therapist who is willing to accept that they may not be optimally knowledgeable or effective will be motivated to learn and to improve.

Before moving on to therapist personal qualities, mention should be made of one last professional characteristic associated with engagement and outcome in psychotherapy: interpersonal skills. One, *empathy*, Rogers (1980) defined as the ability "to perceive the internal frame of reference of another with accuracy and with the emotional components and meanings which pertain thereto as if one were the person" (p. 140). As noted by Norcross and Karpiak (Chapter 5, this volume), "empathic responding is one of the strongest and best supported contributors to psychotherapy outcome" (p. 112). Research reveals it to be the quintessential transdiagnostic and transtheoretical skill. And while therapist assessment of their empathic ability is not reliably associated with actual, measured performance, a series of studies have shown the skill can be improved via a combination of individualized, principle-based feedback and DP (Chow et al., 2022; Miller et al., 2013).

A seminal paradigm for investigating interpersonal skills, known as the Facilitative Interpersonal Skills (FIS) task, was developed by Timothy Anderson and colleagues (https://www.fisresearch.com/research.html). In fact, the studies of empathy just mentioned used a modified version of the FIS rating system. Briefly, the task presents therapists with short video clips of challenging clinical cases (e.g., a client angrily expressing severe disappointment with treatment or strong avoidance and passivity) and records their immediate verbal responses. In turn, independent raters score the responses along several dimensions, encompassing verbal fluency, emotional expressiveness, persuasiveness, warmth, positive regard, hopefulness, empathy, and capacity to repair the working relationship.

Performance on the FIS has been shown to predict treatment outcomes of experienced clinicians of varying orientations, therapist trainees, and even students from nontherapy-related fields who were told merely to "be helpful" (Anderson et al., 2009, 2016). Consistent with the findings on professional discipline, training status (i.e., whether one was learning to be a therapist, biologist, chemist, or historian) does *not* predict performance on the FIS. Confidence in the importance of interpersonal skills is bolstered by results from two additional prospective studies, documenting their ability to predict therapist effectiveness over a 5-year period, even after controlling for myriad therapist (e.g., gender, theoretical orientation, amount of supervision) and client (age, gender, diagnosis, severity, presence of personality disorder) characteristics (Anderson et al., 2016; Schöttke et al., 2017).

Interestingly, experiencing the types of interpersonal challenges reflected on the FIS may be fundamental to the development of personal qualities that matter in effective therapy, such as self-control, emotional containment, and empathy. A recent meta-analysis of 36 studies, for example, found that negative behavioral, cognitive, somatic, and affective therapist reactions toward the client or work are moderately and inversely related to the outcome. Not surprisingly, perhaps, managing such reactions was associated with better results (Hayes et al., 2018).

No section on professional characteristics would be complete without mention of DP. Of course, this entire field guide is devoted to the subject. Despite growing interest and popularity, use of the term in relation to the development of psychotherapists is of recent origin. As reported in Chapter 1, DP was first introduced in a 2007 article by Miller, Hubble, and Duncan to account for therapists who were *consistently* and *significantly* more effective than others (Okiishi et al., 2003; Ricks, 1974). The earliest empirical investigation of the role of DP in the performance of highly effective therapists was carried out by Chow et al. (2015). Consistent with the broader literature on therapist effects, the study involving 69 practitioners and 4,580 clients found (a) clinicians contributed 5.1% to the variance in treatment outcomes, and (b) their age, gender, or caseload were not significant predictors of outcome (see Johns et al., 2019). The main focus of the study, however, was on a subset of the group (17 therapists, 1,632 clients) who completed a measure specifically designed to capture the nature, extent, and time spent in DP activities. Analyses showed that the most effective practitioners devoted 2.8 times more time than their less effective counterparts and 14 times more than those whose outcomes placed them at the bottom of the sample's distribution.

Since the publication of Chow et al. (2015), several prospective studies have appeared in the literature (Di Bartolomeo et al., 2021; Hill et al., 2020; Shukla et al., 2021; Westra et al., 2021). Unfortunately, they fail to meet the four empirically established criteria to qualify as a bona fide instance of DP (i.e., an assessment of the performer's baseline ability or skill level against which progress can be determined, corrective feedback targeted to the individual's execution of skills being learned, development of a plan for successive refinement over time, and guidance provided by an expert coach or teacher; Chow et al., 2015; Ericsson & Lehmann, 1996; Miller et al., 2017, 2018). Accordingly, such studies are best regarded as examples of what Ericsson, the researcher who coined the term *deliberate practice* and conducted the seminal research on the topic, would characterize as "purposeful practice"—repetition aimed at achieving proficiency with a particular skill as opposed to an ongoing process of reaching for performance objectives just beyond an *individual's* current ability (Ericsson, 2016).

There are two exceptions to this. First, a naturalistic study of routine outcome monitoring, feedback, and DP involving more than 5,000 clients and 150 therapists showed small but statistically significant growth in individual clinician effectiveness over time (Goldberg, Babins-Wagner, et al. 2016). According to the authors, the improvement was consistent with findings from the broader DP literature, "highlighting the potentially large cumulative effect of small changes accrued over time" (p. 372). The second, by Chow and colleagues (2022), is the only randomized controlled trial including all four DP components. Designed with guidance and direction from K. Anders Ericsson, the researchers found that therapists employing DP strategies tailored to their specific interpersonal skill deficits not only improved significantly compared with controls (62% vs. 15% gains, respectively), but they also reported that they successfully transferred their newly acquired abilities to different clients, contexts, and clinical themes. By comparison, the control group as a whole—which was instructed to reflect and try to improve on their interpersonal performance scores—did not change appreciably over the course of the study. Importantly, what remains to be documented in future studies is a connection between DP-related skill improvements and gains in outcome at the individual therapist level.

In sum, while promising, much remains unknown about the application of DP to the professional development of psychotherapists. What are the appropriate or most amenable targets (e.g., models, techniques, common contributors to outcome)? How can one best measure the impact (e.g., proximal vs. distal indicators, skill acquisition vs. improvement in treatment outcome, continuous improvement, or proficiency; Miller, Madsen, & Hubble, 2020)? Finally, what role might therapist effects play in the adoption and implementation of DP? Research has already established, for example, that feedback—an essential component of process—is moderated by therapist variables (de Jong et al., 2012). Some of these questions will hopefully be answered as practitioners and researchers investigate, apply, and refine the findings, principles, and exercises recommended in this field guide.

Therapists' Personal Characteristics

Attention is now turned to personal characteristics of therapists—who they are in their private or nonprofessional life, recognizing that distinguishing between the two is sometimes difficult. Myriad qualities could be considered, including values and attitudes, personality, genetic endowment, number of siblings in the family of origin, current level of well-being, quality of life, and job satisfaction, to name but a few. However, this review is limited to the characteristics that have been the subject of research.

To begin, the impacts of several of what might best be labeled "immutable" therapist characteristics have been investigated and found not to contribute to differences in outcome. These characteristics include age, gender, ethnicity, personality constellation, reflective ability, and self-reported social skills (Knox & Hill, 2021). Other more transitory qualities can be added to the list. For example, therapists' self-reported interpersonal problems do not appear to predict their clients' outcomes. Consider the results of a study of over 4,000 clinicians by Heinonen and Orlinsky (2013), which found, across the board, that mental health professionals judged themselves to be *less* accepting and tolerant and *more* critical and demanding in their personal relationships than those with clients. Alas, correspondence between functioning in the personal and professional spheres is not a prerequisite for effectiveness. In their lives outside the consulting room, therapists experience many of the same struggles and pursue many of the same satisfactions for their emotional needs as clients—even if they are trained to put aside those needs in their therapeutic work.

Much attention has been directed to the subject of occupational burnout. Recent evidence indicates that 50% or more of mental health professionals are experiencing moderate levels of emotional exhaustion, depersonalization, and reductions in their sense of accomplishment (Morse et al., 2012; Simionato & Simpson, 2018; Summers et al., 2020). Most—including therapists—would expect such feelings to impact effectiveness negatively. And yet, the evidence is mixed. One large-scale study, for example, found that burnout (specifically *disengagement*—i.e., increased mental distance from work—but not *exhaustion*—i.e., drained, overwhelmed, unable to keep up) and low job satisfaction were associated with poorer treatment outcomes (Delgadillo et al., 2018). However, a more recent investigation conducted in a similar setting found no significant association (Delgadillo et al., 2022).

Given the conflicting results, it is not possible to draw firm conclusions about burnout and client outcomes. However, the research evidence as a whole lends itself to the idea that staying engaged in learning and growing and taking on challenges as a therapist might be beneficial. In a review on the subject, Miller et al. (2015) reported that highly effective therapists experienced lower rates of burnout than average and less effective practitioners. Interestingly, the best therapists also rated *healing involvement* (Orlinsky & Rønnestad, 2005)—the felt sense of being deeply connected to clients—and engagement in traditional self-care practices as *less* important to their work and identity than a focus on results.

In relation to self-care, survey data indicate that therapists generally feel personal therapy is highly influential in their work (Orlinsky et al., 2005). As is true of many of the professional characteristics reviewed here, little empirical evidence exists for an association between personal therapy and performance. Some have suggested experiential practices such as mindfulness activities and self-reflection (Bennett-Levy, 2019) may be helpful for sustaining a career that is emotionally and personally demanding. Notwithstanding, strong support for such practices in terms of measurable outcomes for clients or therapists is thus far lacking.

In terms of other personal qualities, studies have also examined a handful of contemporary concepts. As a predictor of outcome, for example, therapist mindfulness has received mixed results (Hunt et al., 2021; Ivanovic et al., 2015; Pereira et al., 2017; Ryan et al., 2012). Emotional intelligence (EI) has been explored in two investigations. In a small pilot study conducted by Kaplowitz et al. (2011), therapists with higher ratings of EI achieved better therapist-rated outcome results and lower dropout rates compared with therapists with lower ratings of EI. A later, larger study of therapist trainees explored EI in relation to various personality characteristics (e.g., neuroticism, extraversion, openness, agreeableness, and conscientiousness), reporting that the combination of high levels of trainee EI and neuroticism accounted for 46% of the variance in client outcomes (Rieck & Callahan, 2013). While the authors concluded, "EI could be used in determining trainee needs and associated development activities" (Rieck & Callahan, 2013, p. 48), a search of the literature revealed no further publications on the subject.

While investigations of therapists' personal characteristics are few and far between, several have found their impact on outcome varies depending on other client or therapist qualities. So, for instance, while research has generally failed to establish a relationship between outcome and a secure attachment style of the therapist (Petrowski et al., 2011), studies do show such attachment predicts better results for clients with more severe problems (Schauenburg et al., 2010). Similar patterns have been observed in examinations of *reflective functioning*, defined as "the capacity to understand ourselves and others in terms of intentional mental states, such as feelings, desires, wishes, goals and attitudes" (Luyten & Fonagy, 2015, p. 366). To wit, in terms of outcome, higher reflective functioning can compensate for a therapist's attachment-related vulnerabilities and vice versa (i.e., a secure attachment style for deficits in their reflective functioning; Cologon et al., 2017).

In summary, despite an abundance of theory on therapists' personal features, strengths, resources, difficulties, and vulnerabilities, the scientific evidence to date has not yielded replicated support for associations between such features and clinical outcomes (see Table 4.2).

TABLE 4.2. Personal Characteristics and Treatment Outcome

Personal characteristic	Impact on outcome
Age	No correlation
Gender	No correlation
Ethnicity	No correlation
Personal therapy	Little or no evidence of correlation
Big Five personality characteristics	Limited or mixed evidence
Reflective functioning or ability	Promising
Self-reported social skills	No correlation
Therapist reported interpersonal problems	No correlation
Attachment style	Mixed
Mindfulness	Mixed
Burnout	Mixed
Emotional intelligence	Limited evidence

EVIDENCE-BASED PRINCIPLES RELATED TO THERAPIST FACTORS

According to the evidence base summarized in the preceding sections, three principles for DP are most clearly indicated: (a) When in doubt, focus on core interpersonal skills; (b) whatever your model or theoretical approach, be flexible and responsive; and (c) maintain an attitude of humility that supports a willingness to learn and improve. A framework for representing the inter-relationships between these three principles and supporting resources is presented in Figure 4.1.

Principle 1: When in Doubt, Focus on Improving Core Interpersonal Skills

Interpersonal qualities, such as empathy, warmth, and effective communication skills, are the therapist-level characteristics with the most predictive value in terms of positively influencing client outcomes (Heinonen & Nissen-Lie, 2020; Wampold & Owen, 2021). Available evidence shows such skills are trainable (e.g., Anderson et al., 2016). Relatedly, the capacity to tolerate and manage strong negative affect in therapy and stay focused on the emotional state of the client has proven particularly effective when treating clients with higher levels of distress (Heinonen & Nissen-Lie, 2020).

Note that skills and abilities in this area take place at both an external (or expressed) and internal (awareness) level. To function optimally, clinicians need a capacity for *bifurcated* attention, being aware of both the client's and their own 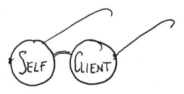 emotional state, containing or regulating any natural but countertherapeutic reactions and responses (see Hayes & Vinca, 2017). Noticing how the client responds to the therapist's interventions—for example, when an empathic and warm response is experienced as intrusive for a client (regardless of what was intended) and evokes withdrawal—offers the opportunity to change tack and initiate repairs. Figure 4.1 displays the relationship between (a) awareness of one's own inner state and countertransference management skills and (b) reflective, perspective taking skills, with both providing essential support for core interpersonal skills (see arrows). It is important to remember that such capacities, research shows, are not gained once and for all. To move beyond mere proficiency, constant work is required across the stages that make up a therapist's career.

Principle 2: Whatever Your Model or Theoretical Approach, Be Flexible and Responsive

Accumulated knowledge in the realm of therapist-level effectiveness indicates that flexibility and responsiveness—adjusting interventions and interactional

FIGURE 4.1. A Framework for Evidence-Based Principles Related to Therapist Factors

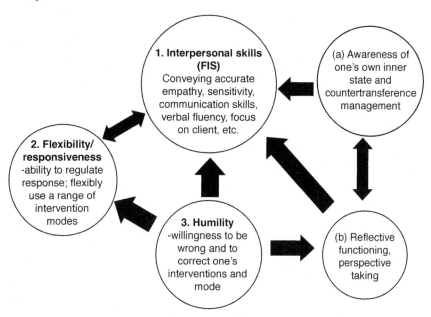

style to the individual client and situation—are key (Constantino et al., 2020; Power et al., 2022; Silberschatz, 2017). Indeed, Stiles and Horvath (2017) argued convincingly, "Certain therapists are more effective than others . . . because [they are] appropriately responsive . . . providing each client with a different, individually tailored treatment" (p. 71).

Over the years, several studies and reviews have indicated that rigid adherence to a model or protocol may hinder the accommodation and tailoring required for working effectively with a given client (see Castonguay et al., 1996; Constantino, Boswell, & Coyne, 2021). Moreover, Owen and Hilsenroth (2014) found that the flexibility therapists demonstrate in the use of techniques within a given treatment—in this case, psychodynamic psychotherapy—was positively related to client improvement. Extending such results, Katz et al. (2019) showed that responding to individual clients by integrating principles from different methods rather than adhering to a set of prescribed principles of one model was also beneficial.

Appropriate *responsiveness* is defined as "behavior that is affected by emerging context, including others' behavior" (Stiles, 2009, p. 87) and should be considered a prerequisite for technical interventions that are useful to the client (see Hatcher, 2015; Stiles & Horvath, 2017). For the therapist, it may be thought of as a metacompetency, tying together a number of lower order skills and capabilities, such as executive functioning, reflection, and interpersonal competencies (Hatcher, 2015). In practical terms, while it might seem difficult to operationalize the concept, a recent metasynthesis of mainly qualitative studies of therapist responsiveness by Wu and Levitt (2020) identified several practical ways therapists could flexibly accommodate their clients, including timing of inter-ventions, affective attunement, attending to underlying relational needs (espe-cially in cases of alliance ruptures or tension), and altering treatment structure and interventions. Turning to specific examples, therapists could check in with the client on a regular basis, be on the lookout for client signals indicating readiness for insight and interpretations, prioritize responding to in-session emotions, as well as employ more directive interventions. In the exercise section that follows, several suggestions are given for DP activities designed to pro-mote flexibility in tailoring one's clinical work to the individual client.

Principle 3: Maintain an Attitude of Humility Supportive of a Willingness to Learn and Improve

In their work and professional development efforts, effective therapists do not avoid conflict or challenging moments. They are open to feedback, seek support from colleagues, and are aware of the demanding nature of psycho-therapy. Humility about one's abilities and effectiveness is not indicative of nor synonymous with performance anxiety or crippling self-doubt; rather, it is a resource that enables therapists to stay alert and remain open to adapting the work to the client. It means truly accepting room *always* exists for growth and pushing beyond one's current skill level, all the while taking care of oneself, including seeking the support needed both personally and professionally to stay on that path.

As Figure 4.1 indicates, humility likely represents the condition (hence the arrows) necessary for the other skills and resources. Without it, the motivation and willingness to learn and improve dissipates. Once more, humility is not about thinking, "I do not know what I'm doing" but rather being open to disconfirming evidence (see Macdonald & Mellor-Clark, 2014; Nissen-Lie et al., 2017). "Could I be wrong?" is a question that opens the door to the devel-opment of expertise. On this score, most practitioners report the process of DP described in the pages of *BR* and this field guide—which emphasizes routinely monitoring the outcome of their work and focusing on one's performance deficits—helps engender that mindset. In the next section, additional sugges-tions in the way of exercises are provided.

EXERCISES FOR THERAPIST FACTOR SKILL DEVELOPMENT

It is often said, "practice makes perfect"; however, that is not necessarily true—practice often simply reinforces habits. Choosing *how* you practice is, therefore, critical. No benefit accrues from engaging in exercises unrelated to your specific pattern of clinical strengths and deficits. To be effective, your DP efforts must be focused on helping you reach for performance objectives just beyond your present abilities. For this reason, before reviewing the following exercises, ensure you have taken all the steps outlined in the decision tree presented

FIELD GUIDE TIP

On the bank of a river, there stood a tall and strong oak tree near to some reeds. The oak tree was proud of its strength and size. He often used to make fun of the weak and slender reeds.

One day, as a wind started blowing, the oak tree, as usual, said mockingly, "Oh! Reeds you move to and fro even with the slightest breeze." The reeds kept quiet and continued to sway back and forth. "Look at me. I am so strong and mighty. Nothing can uproot me or bend me" boasted the oak tree.

The wind got furious and turned into a hurricane. The little reeds prevented themselves from getting uprooted by bowing their heads and swaying with the rhythm of the wind. But the oak tree which stood straight and tried fighting the hurricane wind was soon uprooted and thrown into the river.

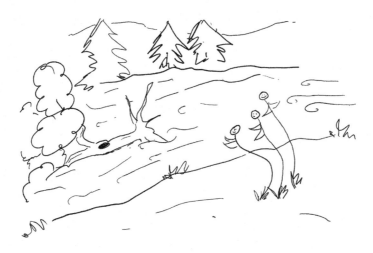

at the start of this chapter. It is assumed you (a) are routinely measuring your performance; (b) have collected sufficient data to establish a reliable, evidence-based profile of your therapeutic effectiveness; (c) completed the TDPA; (d) determined a deficit exists in your performance related to the operation of therapist factors; (e) narrowed your focus to a single element within this domain on the TDPA; and (f) defined that performance improvement objective in SMART terms (specific, measurable, achievable, relevant, and time bound). Next, review the suggested exercises, looking for the one that aligns most closely with your goal.

As you will see, a theme runs through the recommended activities. All are organized around the relationships *between* the evidence-based principles identified from our review of the research as represented in Figure 4.1. This means, for example, applying the various principles (e.g., interpersonal skills, flexibility, responsiveness, humility) in role-play and supervision while simultaneously noting how we feel and actively managing our reactions. Expanding and rehearsing a range of different responses will also prove useful—all the time working at being open and responsive to feedback from the client. Little of the improvement we hope for as therapists comes quickly. Commit to the "long game," setting aside the time to reflect and mentally review your work (Bennett-Levy, 2019). This requires personal reflection and then purposeful action in repetitive practice. As a role model, Miller et al. (2018) offered the example of Pablo Casals, the renowned cellist, who, when questioned as to why even in his later years he practiced for hours each day, responded, "I think I am beginning to show some improvement." Keep in mind that the objective is not perfection, but rather continuous refinement, always being willing to learn and adjust in service of delivering better therapy to clients.

Exercise 1: Who Are You?

Principle: 1
Applicability: TDPA Items 5Ai-iv (also applicable to 3Bi, ii, v, vii, Di-iv, 4B, C, D)
Purpose
As reviewed in detail in *BR*, time and experience within a particular performance domain (e.g., psychotherapy therapy?) lead to the development of "automaticity." While this process enables us to act without having to think through each step we take, the bad news is we lose conscious control over the behaviors mastered. Miller, Hubble, and Chow (2020) observed, "Purposefully counteracting . . . automaticity . . . is at the heart of DP" (p. 28). This exercise is aimed at increasing self-awareness of those automated elements in your interpersonal style and interactions so they can, if needed, be altered.

Task
Part 1. At the end of each day spent meeting with clients, take a few moments to reflect on those sessions you experienced as challenging. With paper and pencil or using your favorite note-keeping software, list the names of the clients, a few identifying characteristics, your "gut" reaction at the time, and your interpersonal response. With regard to the latter, consider the domains on the FIS assessment (e.g., verbal fluency, emotional expressiveness, persuasiveness, warmth, positive regard, hopefulness, empathy, capacity to repair the relationship), rating yourself using a simple Likert rating from 1 to 5. Limit yourself to 20 minutes.

Part 2. After a month, turn your attention to reviewing the information you have gathered, again spending no more than 20 minutes at a time.

- What were your gut reactions?
- What did you feel "pulled" to do with particular clients or situations?

- What, if any, themes and similarities are present (e.g., types of clients, issues, interactions, your responses) across the various sessions described?
- Which aspects of your interpersonal skills suffered the most?

It is important not to rush the process. So, in the time between the moments spent reflecting on your data, resist the temptation to arrive at a firm conclusion. Be mindful, not obsessed with figuring out what to do. Researchers believe that mulling over ideas at length "in the back our minds" has two potential benefits. First, it allows us to make deeper, more nuanced connections between experiences and ideas that, in turn, increase the possibilities for creative action. Second, it influences current behavior, in effect priming us to look for opportunities to act in ways consistent with what we are hoping but presently unable to achieve (e.g., more empathic, less reactive; Wiseman, 2004).

Exercise 2: Civilizing Social Media (or at least trying)

Principle: 1, 3
Applicability: TDPA Items 5Ai–v, viii, 5Bi (also applicable to 3Bi, ii, iv–vi, Di, ii, iv, 4E)
Purpose
Over a relatively brief period, social media have come to occupy a central place in human interactions. Almost half of the world's population is online—3.5 billion people. Two thirds of those use one or more platforms on a regular basis (Ortiz-Ospina, 2019). People get their news, stay in touch with friends and family, connect with like-minded people, watch entertaining videos, and explore their interests. They also argue and fight. In fact, a recent Yale University study found that the algorithms that drive content and connections across various sites actually *teach* users to engage in more hostile and uncivil exchanges (Hathaway, 2021). The frequent occurrence of difficult interactions on these platforms—and the opportunity to reflect for a longer time before responding than would be possible in a real therapeutic interaction—make them the perfect place to practice the types of interpersonal skills associated with effective clinical work.

Task
If you haven't already done so, take some time to familiarize yourself with the literature on interpersonal skills, particularly emotional expressiveness, persuasiveness, warmth, verbal fluency, positive regard, hopefulness, empathy, and capacity to repair the working relationship. Once done, write out your personal definition of each *as well as* several recent instances of their use in interactions with clients.

Next, open your favorite social media app and join a conversation that is either heated or in which the participants are in total agreement with one another. Join in the exchange, mindfully and purposefully using facilitative interpersonal skills to improve engagement openness and civility. Because awareness of your inner state and reactions is critical to responding effectively, take time to reflect before replying to any post or comment made by others. What, if any, feelings are you experiencing? Why? And how do you manage them in the service of maintaining and improving the conversation? Finally, revisit the exchange several times during the week, noting what did and did not work. Regarding the latter, imagine alternate ways you might have responded. Look for any opportunities where you might have been more humble or open to disconfirmation. Continue the exercise indefinitely, slowly ratcheting up the difficulty by seeking out exchanges that are increasingly challenging to your personal beliefs or values.

Exercise 3: Teaching to the Therapeutic Test

Principle: 1, 2
Applicability: TDPA Items 5Aiv, vii, viii (also applicable to 3Bi-iii, v, vi, 3Di, ii)
Purpose
You have likely heard the expression "teaching to the test." This exercise is a variation of that widely discouraged and discredited pedagogical approach! Instead of teaching you to regurgitate the answer you need to improve your performance on a test, this exercise—like all good teaching—is designed to deepen your understanding and use of particular skills. Its origin can be traced to clinicians routinely monitoring their performance with an outcome and alliance scale. Although administered and discussed at the beginning and end of each visit, many reported the tools began to subtly influence how they worked *during* the session. In short, mindful of what clients were being asked to rate, therapists began "doing therapy to the test." Knowing their client would be asked at the end of the visit to rate the degree to which they felt "heard, understood, and respected," for example, encouraged them to reflect on and adjust their responses throughout.

Task
First, open your copy of *BR* and reread Chapter 14, "Designing a System of Deliberate Practice." Second, before each session, quickly review the questions on whatever alliance tool you routinely administer at the end of each visit (e.g., Session Rating Scale; Miller, Duncan, & Johnson, 2000). Even if you have been using the tool for some time and are familiar with its content, don't skip this step. Alternately, write or type out your personal definition of each of the core facilitative interpersonal skills reviewed in this chapter (e.g., emotional expressiveness, persuasiveness, warmth, verbal fluency, positive regard, hopefulness, empathy). Next, pick one to review at the beginning of each session. Importantly, whichever avenue you choose, do not will yourself or make a conscious effort to change what you do in session. Continue with a singular focus on that one interpersonal skill or alliance domain for at least a week.

Third, and finally, the signal you have completed the exercise successfully and can move on to the next can be found at the end of the Exercises section and before Further Reading (see p. 99).

Exercise 4: Seeing Red

Principle: 2
Applicability: TDPA Items 5Ai, ii, iv (also applicable to 1E, F, J, 2D, 4C)
Purpose
Research shows that therapists are not as responsive and flexible with clients who are not progressing or deteriorating in their care. In an analysis of what therapists did in response to such feedback, Lutz (2014) found adjustments in therapeutic interventions were made in less than 30% of cases. In slightly more than 5%, alterations to frequency or intensity and consultations with additional sources of help (e.g., supervision, continuing education, literature review) were made. Clearly, the tendency to "stay the course" is strong. Developing a framework for knowing when and exactly what to do can improve flexibility and responsiveness.

Task
Begin by identifying all completed cases that ended without making progress or dropped out of care. The process is easy if you are using one of the electronic outcome management systems discussed in *BR* (Miller, Hubble, & Chow, 2020). Simply look for clients who ended services in the red zone. It is still possible to do this exercise if you are limited to paper and pencil but just a bit more work. The "Reliable and Clinically Significant Change" chart on page 175 of *BR* (Appendix A) can be used to separate your successful from unsuccessful cases.

Recall, on average, between 24% and 36% of any given therapist's clients end treatment without experiencing a reliable or clinically significant improvement in their well-being or functioning (see Chapter 8 in *BR*). Randomly select 10 such cases, setting aside no more than 30 minutes two or three times a week for in-depth review and analysis. Next, choose one, and with the graph of their outcome scores and your case notes in hand, note the first instance the client was at risk for a negative or null outcome (e.g., entered the red zone, no progress from the prior visit, low or decreasing alliance scores) and what you did in response. For example, did you discuss the results with the client? Adjust your style, approach, interpersonal stance, or dose? Were additional resources suggested, arranged, or consulted? If not, why? If yes, did the client report improvement at the following visit? If not, why? Was it the timing (too much too soon or too little too late)? After exhausting your initial cases, continue the process until a decision tree encompassing the timing of and options for enhanced responsiveness to nonprogressing and "at-risk" clients begins to take shape. Conclude by integrating it into your blueprint (see p. 29 in *BR* and pp. 18–20 in Chapter 1 of this volume).

Exercise 5: Regulating Your Inner Thermometer

Principle: 1
Applicability: TDPA Item 5Ai, ii, iv (also applicable to 3Bi, ii, Di–iv 4C)
Purpose

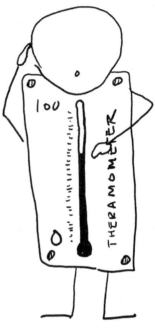

In the practice of Zen, thoughts and emotions are often compared with wind and clouds. They are in constant motion, moving in and out—at times resulting in captivating shapes and scenes and, during others, signaling a storm and the need to take shelter. All are transitory. Enter the terms *cloud* and *Zen* into your favorite search engine, and 20 million hits are returned. The advice offered is strikingly similar across the links: watch and do nothing. Thoughts and emotions, the teachers counsel, are *not* the thinker or person emoting. So, let them float by. No judgment. No connecting. No interpretation. As paradoxical as it may sound, treating thoughts and emotions impersonally—as nothing more than shifting weather patterns—heightens our ability to learn about and better manage our internal world. According to Jon Kabat-Zinn (2019), it enables us to "[make] use of thought and emotion without being caught and imprisoned by unwise and unexamined habit patterns developed over a lifetime" (para. 13).

Doing therapy provokes a wide range of thoughts and emotions. First, there are the feelings and experiences of clients, their hurt, sorrow, fear, anger, guilt, and so on. Second are the thoughts, feelings, and experiences of the therapist—the empathy they feel for those they work with, the joy, frustration, excitement, boredom, discouragement, occasional disgust, and other, sometimes inexplicable, reactions that arise in response to a particular client or their story. As noted in the review of therapist professional characteristics, negative behavioral, cognitive, somatic, and affective reactions toward the client or work are inversely related to the outcome. In short, the greater their number, the less effective the therapy. This exercise is designed to foster awareness and better management of such reactions.

Task

At the end of every few days spent working with clients, reflect on any with whom you experienced a negative cognitive, somatic, and affective reaction. Using a Post-it® note or your favorite note-keeping app, choose one and make a note, listing what you thought or felt, any accompanying physical sensations and their location (e.g., chest, gut, head). As kids are fond of doing with clouds, next, give your reaction a name—maybe the shape or location where it was felt, a person it reminds you of, or a memory. Whether you call it sharp, dull, dog, fish, mountain, stomach, or Bob, do so quickly, without perseverating or looking for hidden meaning. Next, set what you have written aside and spend 5 to 10 minutes quietly and uninterruptedly doing nothing. Whatever happens next, however interesting, foreboding, frightening, or stimulating it may seem, let it pass by like clouds in the sky.

After a month, review your notes, looking for and sorting into patterns. Pay attention to those that recur and elicit the strongest or most disruptive reaction. After refreshing your memory of the particulars, repeat the activity described in the previous paragraph, devoting 5 to 10 minutes to private meditation. You will know progress is being made when you are able to notice quickly but not become absorbed or distracted when "Bob," "sharp," or "mountain" appears.

Exercise 3 Redux: Teaching to the Therapeutic Test

Consistent with the "Playful Experimentations" dimension of the DP framework, you have successfully completed the first round of this exercise *if and when* you spontaneously notice instances of the alliance domain or interpersonal skill you are striving to be mindful of in therapy in activities and experiences *outside* the consulting room (e.g., conversations with family, friends, and colleagues while watching a TV series or movie, in exchanges on social media). If you have not, continue with the same focus for another week.

FURTHER READINGS AND RESOURCES

This chapter reviewed available research, identified evidence-based principles, and suggested DP exercises for working with therapist factors in psychotherapy. Additional research and recommendations can be found in the following:

- The Facilitative Interpersonal Skills (FIS) inventory is a well-validated measure for assessing and improving interpersonal skills. It is available at https://www.fisresearch.com.

- Heinonen, E., & Nissen-Lie, H. (2020). The professional and personal characteristics of effective psychotherapists: A systematic review. *Psychotherapy Research, 30*(4), 417–432. https://doi.org/10.1080/10503307.2019.1620366

- Castonguay, L. G., & Hill, C. E. (2017). *How and why are some therapists better than others? Understanding therapist effects.* American Psychological Association. https://doi.org/10.1037/0000034-000

- Wampold, B. E., & Owen, J. (2021). Therapist effects: History, methods, magnitude, and characteristics of effective therapists. In L. G. Castonguay, M. Barkham, & W. Lutz (Eds.), *Bergin and Garfield's handbook of psychotherapy and behavior change* (7th ed., pp. 301–330). Wiley.

REFERENCES

Anderson, T., McClintock, A. S., Himawan, L., Song, X., & Patterson, C. L. (2016). A prospective study of therapist facilitative interpersonal skills as a predictor of treatment outcome. *Journal of Consulting and Clinical Psychology, 84*(1), 57–66. https://doi.org/10.1037/ccp0000060

Anderson, T., Ogles, B. M., Patterson, C. L., Lambert, M. J., & Vermeersch, D. A. (2009). Therapist effects: Facilitative interpersonal skills as a predictor of therapist success. *Journal of Clinical Psychology, 65*(7), 755–768. https://doi.org/10.1002/jclp.20583

Baldwin, S. A., & Imel, Z. (2013). Therapist effects. In M. J. Lambert (Ed.), *Bergin and Garfield's handbook of psychotherapy and behavior change* (6th ed., pp. 258–297). Wiley.

Barkham, M., & Lambert, M. J. (2021). The efficacy and effectiveness of psychological therapies. In M. Barkham, W. Lutz, & L. G. Castonguay (Eds.), *Bergin & Garfield's handbook of psychotherapy and behavior change.* (7th ed., pp. 135–190). Wiley.

Barkham, M., Lutz, W., Lambert, M. J., & Saxon, D. (2017). Therapist effects, effective therapists, and the law of variability. In L. G. Castonguay & C. E. Hill (Eds.), *How and why are some therapists better than others? Understanding therapist effects* (pp. 13–36). American Psychological Association. https://doi.org/10.1037/0000034-002

Bennett-Levy, J. (2019). Why therapists should walk the talk: The theoretical and empirical case for personal practice in therapist training and professional development. *Journal of Behavior Therapy and Experimental Psychiatry, 62,* 133–145. https://doi.org/10.1016/j.jbtep.2018.08.004

Beutler, L. E., Malik, M., Alimohamed, S., Harwood, T. M., Talebi, H., Noble, S., & Wong, E. (2004). Therapist variables. In M. J. Lambert (Ed.), *Bergin and Garfield's handbook of psychotherapy and behavior change* (5th ed., pp. 227–306). Wiley.

Castonguay, L. G., Goldfried, M. R., Wiser, S., Raue, P. J., & Hayes, A. M. (1996). Predicting the effect of cognitive therapy for depression: A study of unique and common factors. *Journal of Consulting and Clinical Psychology, 64*(3), 497–504. https://doi.org/10.1037/0022-006X.64.3.497

Castonguay, L. G., & Hill, C. E. (Eds.). (2017). *How and why are some therapists better than others? Understanding therapist effects.* American Psychological Association. https://doi.org/10.1037/0000034-000

Chow, D., Lu, S., Miller, S., Kwek, T., Jones, A., & Hubble, M. (2022). *Improving difficult conversations in therapy: A randomized trial of a deliberate practice training program* [Manuscript submitted for publication]. International Center for Clinical Excellence, Chicago, IL.

Chow, D., & Miller, S. D. (2022). *Taxonomy of Deliberate Practice Activities in Psychotherapy—Therapist Version* (Version 6). International Center for Clinical Excellence.

Chow, D. L., Miller, S. D., Seidel, J. A., Kane, R. T., Thornton, J. A., & Andrews, W. P. (2015). The role of deliberate practice in the development of highly effective psychotherapists. *Psychotherapy, 52*(3), 337–345. https://doi.org/10.1037/pst0000015

Cologon, J., Schweitzer, R. D., King, R., & Nolte, T. (2017). Therapist reflective functioning, therapist attachment style and therapist effectiveness. *Administration and Policy in Mental Health, 44*(5), 614–625. https://doi.org/10.1007/s10488-017-0790-5

Constantino, M. J., Boswell, F. J., & Coyne, A. E. (2021). Patient, therapist, and relational factors. In M. Barkham, W. Lutz, & L. G. Castonguay (Eds.), *Bergin and Garfield's handbook of psychotherapy and behavior change* (7th ed., pp. 225–262). Wiley.

Constantino, M. J., Boswell, J. F., Coyne, A. E., Swales, T. P., & Kraus, D. R. (2021). Effect of matching therapists to patients vs assignment as usual on adult psychotherapy outcomes: A randomized clinical trial. *JAMA Psychiatry, 78*(9), 960–969. https://doi.org/10.1001/jamapsychiatry.2021.1221

Constantino, M. J., Coyne, A. E., & Muir, H. J. (2020). Evidence-based therapist responsivity to disruptive clinical process. *Cognitive and Behavioral Practice, 27*(4), 405–416. https://doi.org/10.1016/j.cbpra.2020.01.003

Crits-Christoph, P., Baranackie, K., Kurcias, J. S., Beck, A. T., Carroll, K., Perry, K., Luborsky, L., McLellan, A., Woody, G., Thompson, L., Gallagher, D., & Zitrin, C. (1991). Meta-analysis of therapist effects in psychotherapy outcome studies. *Psychotherapy Research, 1*(2), 81–91. https://doi.org/10.1080/10503309112331335511

de Jong, K., van Sluis, P., Nugter, M. A., Heiser, W. J., & Spinhoven, P. (2012). Understanding the differential impact of outcome monitoring: Therapist variables that moderate feedback effects in a randomized clinical trial. *Psychotherapy Research, 22*(4), 464–474. https://doi.org/10.1080/10503307.2012.673023

Delgadillo, J., Nissen-Lie, H. A., de Jong, K., Schröder, T. A., & Barkham, M. (2022). *Therapist effects in a randomised controlled trial of feedback-informed psychological treatment for depression and anxiety* [Manuscript in preparation]. Clinical and Applied Psychology Unit, University of Sheffield.

Delgadillo, J., Rubel, J., & Barkham, M. (2020). Towards personalized allocation of patients to therapists. *Journal of Consulting and Clinical Psychology, 88*(9), 799–808. https://doi.org/10.1037/ccp0000507

Delgadillo, J., Saxon, D., & Barkham, M. (2018). Associations between therapists' occupational burnout and their patients' depression and anxiety treatment outcomes. *Depression and Anxiety, 35*(9), 844–850. https://doi.org/10.1002/da.22766

Di Bartolomeo, A. A., Shukla, S., Westra, H. A., Shekarak Ghashghaei, N., & Olson, D. A. (2021). Rolling with resistance: A client language analysis of deliberate practice in continuing education for psychotherapists. *Counselling & Psychotherapy Research, 21*(2), 433–441. https://doi.org/10.1002/capr.12335

Edmondstone, C., Pascual-Leone, A., Soucie, K., & Kramer, U. (2022). Therapist effects on outcome: Meaningful differences exist early in training. *Training and Education in Professional Psychology.* Advance online publication. https://doi.org/10.1037/tep0000402

Ericsson, K. A. (2016). Summing up hours of any type of practice versus identifying optimal practice activities: Commentary on Macnamara, Moreau, and Hambrick (2016). *Perspectives on Psychological Science, 11*(3), 351–354. https://doi.org/10.1177/1745691616635600

Ericsson, K. A., & Lehmann, A. G. (1996). Expert and exceptional performance: Evidence of maximal adaptation to task constraints. *Annual Review of Psychology, 47*(1), 273–305. https://doi.org/10.1146/annurev.psych.47.1.273

Firth, N., Barkham, M., Kellett, S., & Saxon, D. (2015). Therapist effects and moderators of effectiveness and efficiency in psychological wellbeing practitioners: A multilevel modelling analysis. *Behaviour Research and Therapy, 69*, 54–62. https://doi.org/10.1016/j.brat.2015.04.001

Frank, J. D. (1961). *Persuasion and healing: A comparative study of psychotherapy.* Johns Hopkins University Press.

Frank, J. D., & Frank, J. B. (1991). *Persuasion and healing: A comparative study of psychotherapy* (3rd ed.). Johns Hopkins University Press.

Goldberg, S. B., Babins-Wagner, R., Rousmaniere, T., Berzins, S., Hoyt, W. T., Whipple, J. L., Miller, S. D., & Wampold, B. E. (2016). Creating a climate for therapist improvement: A case study of an agency focused on outcomes and deliberate practice. *Psychotherapy, 53*(3), 367–375. https://doi.org/10.1037/pst0000060

Goldberg, S. B., Rousmaniere, T., Miller, S. D., Whipple, J., Nielsen, S. L., Hoyt, W. T., & Wampold, B. E. (2016). Do psychotherapists improve with time and experience? A longitudinal analysis of outcomes in a clinical setting. *Journal of Counseling Psychology, 63*(1), 1–11. https://doi.org/10.1037/cou0000131

Hatcher, R. L. (2015). Interpersonal competencies: Responsiveness, technique, and training in psychotherapy. *American Psychologist, 70*(8), 747–757. https://doi.org/10.1037/a0039803

Hathaway, B. (2021, August 13). 'Likes' and 'shares' teach people to express more outrage online. *Yale News.* https://news.yale.edu/2021/08/13/likes-and-shares-teach-people-express-more-outrage-online

Hayes, J. A., Gelso, C. J., Goldberg, S., & Kivlighan, D. M. (2018). Countertransference management and effective psychotherapy: Meta-analytic findings. *Psychotherapy*, 55(4), 496–507. https://doi.org/10.1037/pst0000189

Hayes, J. A., McAleavey, A. A., Castonguay, L. G., & Locke, B. D. (2016). Psychotherapists' outcomes with White and racial/ethnic minority clients: First, the good news. *Journal of Counseling Psychology*, 63(3), 261–268. https://doi.org/10.1037/cou0000098

Hayes, J. A., & Vinca, M. (2017). Therapist presence, absence and extraordinary presence. In L. G. Castonguay & C. E. Hill (Eds.), *How and why are some therapists better than others? Understanding therapist effects* (pp. 85–99). American Psychological Association. https://doi.org/10.1037/0000034-006

Heinonen, E., & Nissen-Lie, H. A. (2020). The professional and personal characteristics of effective psychotherapists: A systematic review. *Psychotherapy Research*, 30(4), 417–432. https://doi.org/10.1080/10503307.2019.1620366

Heinonen, E., & Orlinsky, D. E. (2013). Psychotherapists' personal identities, theoretical orientations, and professional relationships: Elective affinity and role adjustment as modes of congruence. *Psychotherapy Research*, 23(6), 718–731. https://doi.org/10.1080/10503307.2013.814926

Hill, C. E., Kivlighan, D. M., III, Rousmaniere, T., Kivlighan, D. M., Jr., Gerstenblith, J. A., & Hillman, J. W. (2020). Deliberate practice for the skill of immediacy: A multiple case study of doctoral student therapists and clients. *Psychotherapy*, 57(4), 587–597. https://doi.org/10.1037/pst0000247

Hunt, C., Goodman, R., Hilert, A., Hurley, W., & Hill, C. (2021). A mindfulness-based compassion workshop and pre-session preparation to enhance therapist effectiveness in psychotherapy: A pilot study. *Counselling Psychology Quarterly*. Advance online publication. https://doi.org/10.1080/09515070.2021.1895724

Imel, Z. E., Baldwin, S., Atkins, D. C., Owen, J., Baardseth, T., & Wampold, B. E. (2011). Racial/ethnic disparities in therapist effectiveness: A conceptualization and initial study of cultural competence. *Journal of Counseling Psychology*, 58(3), 290–298. https://doi.org/10.1037/a0023284

Ivanovic, M., Swift, J. K., Callahan, J. L., & Dunn, R. (2015). A multisite pre/post study of mindfulness training for therapists: The impact on session presence and effectiveness. *Journal of Cognitive Psychotherapy*, 29(4), 331–342. https://doi.org/10.1891/0889-8391.29.4.331

Johns, R. G., Barkham, M., Kellett, S., & Saxon, D. (2019). A systematic review of therapist effects: A critical narrative update and refinement to review. *Clinical Psychology Review*, 67, 78–93. https://doi.org/10.1016/j.cpr.2018.08.004

Kabat-Zinn, J. (2019, March 20). A meditation on observing thoughts, non-judgmentally. *Mindful: Healthy Mind, Healthy Life*. https://www.mindful.org/a-meditation-on-observing-thoughts-non-judgmentally/

Kaplowitz, M. J., Safran, J. D., & Muran, C. J. (2011). Impact of therapist emotional intelligence on psychotherapy. *Journal of Nervous and Mental Disease*, 199(2), 74–84. https://doi.org/10.1097/NMD.0b013e3182083efb

Katz, M., Hilsenroth, M. J., Gold, J. R., Moore, M., Pitman, S. R., Levy, S. R., & Owen, J. (2019). Adherence, flexibility, and outcome in psychodynamic treatment of depression. *Journal of Counseling Psychology*, 66(1), 94–103. https://doi.org/10.1037/cou0000299

Knox, S., & Hill, C. (2021). Training and supervision in psychotherapy: What we know and where we need to go. In M. Barkham, W. Lutz, & L. G. Castonguay (Eds.), *Bergin and Garfield's handbook of psychotherapy and behavior change* (7th ed., pp. 327–350). Wiley.

Kraus, D. R., Castonguay, L., Boswell, J. F., Nordberg, S. S., & Hayes, J. A. (2011). Therapist effectiveness: Implications for accountability and patient care. *Psychotherapy Research*, 21(3), 267–276. https://doi.org/10.1080/10503307.2011.563249

Lutz, W. (2014, December). *Why, when, and how do patients change? Identifying and predict-ing progress and outcome in psychotherapy.* https://www.scottdmiller.com/wp-content/uploads/2016/09/Lecture-Wolfgang-Lutz-Calgary2014_send.pdf

Lutz, W., Rubel, J., Schiefele, A. K., Zimmermann, D., Böhnke, J. R., & Wittmann, W. W. (2015). Feedback and therapist effects in the context of treatment outcome and treatment length. *Psychotherapy Research, 25*(6), 647–660. https://doi.org/10.1080/10503307.2015.1053553

Luyten, P., & Fonagy, P. (2015). The neurobiology of mentalizing. *Personality Disorders, 6*(4), 366–379. https://doi.org/10.1037/per0000117.

Macdonald, J., & Mellor-Clark, J. (2014). Correcting psychotherapists' blindsidedness: Formal feedback as a means of overcoming the natural limitations of therapists. *Clinical Psychology & Psychotherapy, 22*(3), 249–257. https://doi.org/10.1002/cpp.1887

Miller, S. D., Chow, D., Wampold, B., Hubble, M. A., Del Re, A. C., Maeschalck, C., & Bargmann, S. (2018). To be or not to be (an expert)? Revisiting the role of deliberate practice in improving performance. *High Ability Studies, 31*(1), 5–15. https://doi.org/10.1080/13598139.2018.1519410

Miller, S. D., Duncan, B. L., & Johnson, L. D. (2000). *The Session Rating Scale 3.0.* Inter-national Center for Clinical Excellence.

Miller, S. D., Hubble, M. A., & Chow, D. (2020). *Better results: Using deliberate practice to improve therapeutic effectiveness.* American Psychological Association. https://doi.org/10.1037/0000191-000

Miller, S. D., Hubble, M. A., Chow, D. L., & Seidel, J. A. (2013). The outcome of psycho-therapy: Yesterday, today, and tomorrow. *Psychotherapy, 50*(1), 88–97. https://doi.org/10.1037/a0031097

Miller, S. D., Hubble, M. A., & Mathieu, F. (2015, May–June). Burnout reconsidered. *Psychotherapy Networker, 39*(3), 18–23, 42–43.

Miller, S. D., Hubble, M. A., & Wampold, B. E. (2017). Growing better therapists: A new opportunity for mental health administrators. *Administration and Policy in Mental Health, 44*(5), 732–734. https://doi.org/10.1007/s10488-017-0805-2

Miller, S. D., Madsen, J., & Hubble, M. A. (2020). Toward an evidence-based standard of professional competence. In M. Trachsel, J. Gaab, N. Biller-Andorno, S. Tekin, & J. Sadler (Eds.), *Oxford handbook of psychotherapy ethics* (pp. 951–968). Oxford University Press.

Morse, G., Salyers, M. P., Rollins, A. L., Monroe-DeVita, M., & Pfahler, C. (2012). Burnout in mental health services: A review of the problem and its remediation. *Administration and Policy in Mental Health, 39*(5), 341–352. https://doi.org/10.1007/s10488-011-0352-1

Nissen-Lie, H. A., Goldberg, S. B., Hoyt, W. T., Falkenström, F., Holmqvist, R., Nielsen, S. L., & Wampold, B. E. (2016). Are therapists uniformly effective across patient outcome domains? A study on therapist effectiveness in two different treatment contexts. *Journal of Counseling Psychology, 63*(4), 367–378. https://doi.org/10.1037/cou0000151

Nissen-Lie, H. A., Monsen, J. T., & Rønnestad, M. H. (2010). Therapist predictors of early patient-rated working alliance: A multilevel approach. *Psychotherapy Research, 20*(6), 627–646. https://doi.org/10.1080/10503307.2010.497633

Nissen-Lie, H. A., Monsen, J. T., Ulleberg, P., & Rønnestad, M. H. (2013). Psychothera-pists' self-reports of their interpersonal functioning and difficulties in practice as predictors of patient outcome. *Psychotherapy Research, 23*(1), 86–104. https://doi.org/10.1080/10503307.2012.735775

Nissen-Lie, H. A., Rønnestad, M. H., Høglend, P. A., Havik, O. E., Solbakken, O. A., Stiles, T. C., & Monsen, J. T. (2017). Love yourself as a person, doubt yourself as a therapist? *Clinical Psychology & Psychotherapy, 24*(1), 48–60. https://doi.org/10.1002/cpp.1977

Odyniec, P., Probst, T., Margraf, J., & Willutzki, U. (2019). Psychotherapist trainees' professional self-doubt and negative personal reaction: Changes during cognitive behavioral therapy and association with patient progress. *Psychotherapy Research*, *29*(1), 123–138. https://doi.org/10.1080/10503307.2017.1315464

Okiishi, J., Lambert, M. J., Nielsen, S. L., & Ogles, B. M. (2003). Waiting for supershrink: An empirical analysis of therapist effects. *Clinical Psychology & Psychotherapy, 10*(6), 361–373. https://doi.org/10.1002/cpp.383

Orlinsky, D. E., Norcross, J. C., Rønnestad, M. H., & Wiseman, H. (2005). Outcomes and impacts of the psychotherapists' own psychotherapy: A research review. In J. D. Geller, J. C. Norcross, & D. E. Orlinsky (Eds.), *The psychotherapist's own psychotherapy: Patient and clinician perspectives* (pp. 214–235). Oxford University Press.

Orlinsky, D. E., & Rønnestad, M. H. (2005). *How psychotherapists develop: A study of therapeutic work and professional growth.* American Psychological Association. https://doi.org/10.1037/11157-000

Ortiz-Ospina, E. (2019). The rise of social media. *Our world in data.* https://ourworldindata.org/rise-of-social-media

Owen, J., Drinane, J. M., Idigo, K. C., & Valentine, J. C. (2015). Psychotherapist effects in meta-analyses: How accurate are treatment effects? *Psychotherapy, 52*(3), 321–328. https://doi.org/10.1037/pst0000014

Owen, J., Drinane, J. M., Kivlighan, M., Miller, S., Kopta, M., & Imel, Z. (2019). Are high-performing therapists both effective and consistent? A test of therapist expertise. *Journal of Consulting and Clinical Psychology, 87*(12), 1149–1156. https://doi.org/10.1037/ccp0000437

Owen, J., & Hilsenroth, M. J. (2014). Treatment adherence: The importance of therapist flexibility in relation to therapy outcomes. *Journal of Counseling Psychology, 61*(2), 280–288. https://doi.org/10.1037/a0035753

Pereira, J. A., Barkham, M., Kellett, S., & Saxon, D. (2017). The role of practitioner resilience and mindfulness in effective practice: A practice-based feasibility study. *Administration and Policy in Mental Health, 44*(5), 691–704. https://doi.org/10.1007/s10488-016-0747-0

Petrowski, K., Nowacki, K., Pokorny, D., & Buchheim, A. (2011). Matching the patient to the therapist: The roles of the attachment status and the helping alliance. *Journal of Nervous and Mental Disease, 199*(11), 839–844. https://doi.org/10.1097/NMD.0b013e3182349cce

Power, N., Noble, L. A., Simmonds-Buckley, M., Kellett, S., Stockton, C., Firth, N., & Delgadillo, J. (2022). Associations between treatment adherence-competence-integrity (ACI) and adult psychotherapy outcomes: A systematic review and meta-analysis. *Journal of Consulting and Clinical Psychology, 90*(5), 427–445. https://doi.org/10.1037/ccp0000736

Ricks, D. F. (1974). Supershrink: Methods of a therapist judged successful on the basis of adult outcomes of adolescent patients. In D. F. Ricks, M. Roff, & A. Thomas (Eds.), *Life history research in psychopathology* (Vol. 3, pp. 275–297). University of Minnesota Press.

Rieck, T., & Callahan, J. L. (2013). Emotional intelligence and psychotherapy outcomes in the training clinic. *Training and Education in Professional Psychology, 7*(1), 42–52. https://doi.org/10.1037/a0031659

Rogers, C. R. (1957). The necessary and sufficient conditions of therapeutic personality change. *Journal of Consulting Psychology, 21*(2), 95–103. https://doi.org/10.1037/h0045357

Rogers, C. R. (1980). *A way of being.* Houghton Mifflin.

Rosenzweig, S. (1936). Some implicit common factors in diverse methods of psychotherapy. *American Journal of Orthopsychiatry, 6*(3), 412–415. https://doi.org/10.1111/j.1939-0025.1936.tb05248.x

Roth, A. D., & Pilling, S. (2008). Using an evidence-based methodology to identify the competences required to deliver effective cognitive and behavioural therapy for depression and anxiety disorders. *Behavioural and Cognitive Psychotherapy, 36*(2), 129–147. https://doi.org/10.1017/S1352465808004141

Ryan, A., Safran, J. D., Doran, J. M., & Muran, J. C. (2012). Therapist mindfulness, alliance and treatment outcome. *Psychotherapy Research, 22*(3), 289–297. https://doi.org/10.1080/10503307.2011.650653

Saxon, D., & Barkham, M. (2012). Patterns of therapist variability: Therapist effects and the contribution of patient severity and risk. *Journal of Consulting and Clinical Psychology, 80*(4), 535–546. https://doi.org/10.1037/a0028898

Schauenburg, H., Buchheim, A., Beckh, K., Nolte, T., Brenk-Franz, K., Leichsenring, F., Strack, M., & Dinger, U. (2010). The influence of psychodynamically oriented therapists' attachment representations on outcome and alliance in inpatient psychotherapy [corrected]. *Psychotherapy Research, 20*(2), 193–202. https://doi.org/10.1080/10503300903204043

Schöttke, H., Flückiger, C., Goldberg, S. B., Eversmann, J., & Lange, J. (2017). Predicting psychotherapy outcome based on therapist interpersonal skills: A five-year longitudinal study of a therapist assessment protocol. *Psychotherapy Research, 27*(6), 642–652. https://doi.org/10.1080/10503307.2015.1125546

Shukla, S., Di Bartolomeo, A. A., Westra, H. A., Olson, D. A., & Shekarak Ghashghaei, N. (2021). The impact of a deliberate practice workshop on therapist demand and support behavior with community volunteers and simulators. *Psychotherapy, 58*(2), 186–195. https://doi.org/10.1037/pst0000333

Silberschatz, G. (2017). Improving the yield of psychotherapy research. *Psychotherapy Research, 27*(1), 1–13. https://doi.org/10.1080/10503307.2015.1076202

Simionato, G. K., & Simpson, S. (2018). Personal risk factors associated with burnout among psychotherapists: A systematic review of the literature. *Journal of Clinical Psychology, 74*(9), 1431–1456. https://doi.org/10.1002/jclp.22615

Stiles, W. B. (2009). Responsiveness as an obstacle for psychotherapy outcome research: It's worse than you think. *Clinical Psychology: Science and Practice, 16*(1), 86–91. https://doi.org/10.1111/j.1468-2850.2009.01148.x

Stiles, W. B., & Horvath, A. O. (2017). Appropriate responsiveness as a contribution to therapist effects. In L. G. Castonguay & C. E. Hill (Eds.), *How and why are some therapists better than others? Understanding therapist effects* (pp. 71–84). American Psychological Association. https://doi.org/10.1037/0000034-005

Summers, R. F., Gorrindo, T., Hwang, S., Aggarwal, R., & Guille, C. (2020). Well-being, burnout, and depression among north American psychiatrists: The state of our profession. *The American Journal of Psychiatry, 177*(10), 955–964. Advance online publication. https://doi.org/10.1176/appi.ajp.2020.19090901

Walfish, S., McAlister, B., O'Donnell, P., & Lambert, M. J. (2012). An investigation of self-assessment bias in mental health providers. *Psychological Reports, 110*(2), 639–644. https://doi.org/10.2466/02.07.17.PR0.110.2.639-644

Wampold, B. E. (2001). *The great psychotherapy debate: Models, methods, and findings.* Erlbaum.

Wampold, B. E., & Brown, G. S. (2005). Estimating variability in outcomes attributable to therapists: A naturalistic study of outcomes in managed care. *Journal of Consulting and Clinical Psychology, 73*(5), 914–923. https://doi.org/10.1037/0022-006X.73.5.914

Wampold, B. E., & Imel, Z. E. (2015). *The great psychotherapy debate: The evidence for what works in psychotherapy.* Routledge. https://doi.org/10.4324/9780203582015

Wampold, B. E., & Owen, J. (2021). Therapist effects: History, methods, magnitude, and characteristics of effective therapists. In M. Barkham, W. Lutz, & L. G. Castonguay (Eds.), *Bergin and Garfield's handbook of psychotherapy and behavior change* (7th ed., pp. 301–330). Wiley.

Webb, C. A., Derubeis, R. J., & Barber, J. P. (2010). Therapist adherence/competence and treatment outcome: A meta-analytic review. *Journal of Consulting and Clinical Psychology*, *78*(2), 200–211. https://doi.org/10.1037/a0018912

Westra, H. A., Norouzian, N., Poulin, L., Coyne, A., Constantino, M. J., Hara, K., Olson, D., & Antony, M. M. (2021). Testing a deliberate practice workshop for developing appropriate responsivity to resistance markers. *Psychotherapy: Theory, Research, & Practice*, *58*(2), 175–185. https://doi.org/10.1037/pst0000311

Wiseman, R. (2004). *Did you spot the gorilla?* Arrow.

Wu, M. B., & Levitt, H. M. (2020). A qualitative meta-analytic review of the therapist responsiveness literature: Guidelines for practice and training. *Journal of Contemporary Psychotherapy*, *50*(3), 161–175. https://doi.org/10.1007/s10879-020-09450-y

Ziede, J. S., & Norcross, J. C. (2020). Personal therapy and self-care in the making of psychologists. *The Journal of Psychology*, *154*(8), 585–618. https://doi.org/10.1080/00223980.2020.1757596

Ziem, M., & Hoyer, J. (2020). Modest, yet progressive: Effective therapists tend to rate therapeutic change less positively than their patients. *Psychotherapy Research*, *30*(4), 433–446. https://doi.org/10.1080/10503307.2019.1631502

5

Relationship Factors

John C. Norcross and Christie P. Karpiak

We are born in relationship, we are wounded in relationship, and we can be healed in relationship.

—HARVILLE HENDRIX, *GETTING THE LOVE YOU WANT*

DECISION POINT

Begin here if you have read the book *Better Results* and

- are routinely measuring your performance *and*
- have collected sufficient data to establish a reliable, evidence-based profile of your therapeutic effectiveness *and*
- have completed the Taxonomy of Deliberate Practice Activities in Psychotherapy *and*
- need help developing deliberate practice exercises related to relationship factors.

Second only to the client's contribution, the psychotherapy relationship is the most important predictor of, and contributor to, outcome. The relationship constitutes the heart and soul of psychotherapy, healing in and of itself. Even when offered as a manualized intervention and delivered via electronic means, it is invariably rooted in and dependent on that complex connection

https://doi.org/10.1037/0000358-006
The Field Guide to Better Results: Evidence-Based Exercises to Improve Therapeutic Effectiveness,
S. D. Miller, D. Chow, S. Malins, and M. A. Hubble (Editors)

between the client and therapist. As such, it warrants substantial attention as part of deliberate practice (DP).

There is little clinicians can do to directly alter most preexisting client factors or events in clients' lives outside the session. The relationship, however, is curated and cultivated by the therapist's attitudes and behaviors from the first moments of contact. On this score, the evidence shows clinicians differ in their ability to facilitate effective therapeutic connections (Castonguay & Hill, 2017; Norcross & Wampold, 2019), and their capacity can be developed and improved through monitoring, training, and practice. Importantly, the efficacy of these relationship factors cuts across theoretical orientations (transtheoretical) and largely across client problems (transdiagnostic). The factors considered in this chapter—the alliance, collaboration, goal consensus, empathy, positive regard/affirmation, congruence/genuineness, emotional expression, and repairing alliance ruptures—have all been shown, in dozens of individual studies and in rigorous meta-analyses, to associate, predict, and contribute to success. Failure to provide these elements also predicts and contributes to poor results, however measured (e.g., dropout, deterioration).

Why would any responsible mental health professional deliberately practice behaviors of unknown, dubious, or no association with psychotherapy success? Yet, many routinely do so. A case in point can be found in the practice of "confronting" clients. While it may prove a crowd-pleaser for talk-show therapists, it corresponds with poor therapy outcome—even in treatment areas like addictions, where there remains some belief that it is a good way for therapists to behave (W. R. Miller, 2018; W. R. Miller & Rollnick, 2012). Ethics and evidence demand those behaviors that demonstrably work be taught, practiced, and employed in care. And these evidence-based relational factors do just that. Indeed, given their significant contribution, it is hard to imagine a better focus for DP than establishing responsive and respectful relationships.

Before proceeding, it is important to define the terms and register a few conceptual caveats regarding the material that follows. An operational definition of the *therapeutic relationship* is the feelings and attitudes that therapist and client have toward one another and the manner in which these are expressed (Gelso & Carter, 1985, 1994). While this definition is quite general, it is concise, consensual, theoretically neutral, and sufficiently precise.

The frequently used term *therapeutic alliance* represents a part of the relationship, but only a part. In fact, a pernicious error in the psychotherapy literature equates the totality of the relationship with the therapeutic alliance. In part, this mistake occurs inadvertently because the alliance is the most frequently measured and researched relationship factor in the psychotherapy literature (Horvath et al., 2016). However, it is also intentional, an effort to misrepresent and diminish the cumulative power of the relationship. Ironically, the alliance's association with psychotherapy success is not even the largest of the relationship factors. That distinction, as will be shown, resides with empathy (see Table 5.2). In reality, the alliance accounts for less treatment outcome than the many relationship behaviors research shows are demonstrably effective (Norcross & Lambert, 2019). Thus, confounding the entirety of the therapy

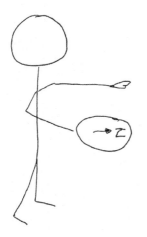

FIELD GUIDE TIP

Keep in mind: The relationship is more than agreement on goals, tasks, and provision of the Rogerian core conditions. It actually includes a genuine liking of the client!

relationship with only the alliance weakens the power of the therapeutic relationship empirically and clinically.

There are several other caveats to consider. First, the relationship factors reviewed in this chapter are not independent of one another. They are inherently interrelated, and it is likely many or most happen together in effective therapy and fail together in a poor one (Nienhuis et al., 2018; Watson & Geller, 2005). Second, the boundaries among the elements described in this chapter, and those presented in others, are fuzzy rather than distinct and mutually exclusive. For instance, therapist responsiveness or personalization (Norcross & Cooper, 2021; Norcross & Wampold, 2019)—a powerful contributor to effectiveness—is connected to relationship, client, *and* therapist factors (see Chapters 3 and 4, this volume). Third, this review is focused on the contribution of relationship factors to the outcome of individual psychotherapy, although the evidence is equally compelling for its power in couple, family, and group therapy (Burlingame et al., 2019; Friedlander et al., 2019), as well as pharmacotherapy (Totura et al., 2018).

As a field guide, this book is designed to be practical in nature, focusing on strategy rather than theory. Such pragmatism informs this chapter, including the review of the empirical research, the identification of evidence-based principles, and the recommended DP exercises. With regard to the latter, the majority are specifically designed to assist practitioners in addressing deficits in their therapeutic relationships, not achieving brilliance. After all, practice does not make perfect; it is the adjustments and refinements that follow from practice (Ripken, 2019).

REVIEW OF THE RESEARCH

Empirical research on the therapeutic relationship spans more than half a century. Originally considered primarily in psychodynamic and humanistic therapies, decades ago, it became evident relationship factors are potent regardless of theoretical model or modality. Scholarly reviews of transtheoretical therapeutic factors (i.e., "common factors"), including the relationship, appeared in edition after edition of the *Handbook of Psychotherapy and Behavior Change* (Lambert & Hill, 1994; Orlinsky et al., 1994). Starting in 2002, the vast accumulated evidence specifically in support of relationship factors was presented in Norcross's *Psychotherapy Relationships That Work*. The most recent, published in two volumes, compiles meta-analyses of more than 15 relationship factors (Norcross & Lambert, 2019; Norcross & Wampold, 2019). These studies, also truncated and reported in special journal issues, are the source of the effect sizes reported in Table 5.2. Simply put, no scientific doubt exists about the contribution of the relationship to outcome. Neither is there any doubt that the relationship is more determinative for results than the treatment model or type (Wampold & Imel, 2015).

Part of the reason for the contemporary emphasis on learning treatment packages has been the misconception that, while specific treatments can be taught, the ability to form therapeutic relationships is both ethereal and fixed. Recent reviews should forever put such notions and claims to rest (e.g., Knox & Hill, 2021). The relationship might be part of the "art" of psychotherapy, but most of its effective components are definable, measurable, and learnable. In other words, relational abilities are not immutable (Anderson et al., 2020). While some therapists are better than others at facilitating and maintaining effective connections, others can learn and improve on those skills. Indeed, there would be little point in including this chapter in the *Field Guide* (*FG*) were that not the case.

Relationship Factors That Do *Not* Make a Difference

Translational research is both prescriptive and proscriptive; it tells us what works and what does not. In this section, ineffective, perhaps even hurtful, therapist relational behaviors are highlighted (see Table 5.1; Norcross & Lambert, 2019). One means of identifying such qualities is simply to reverse the effective behaviors identified in the meta-analyses reviewed in the next section. Thus, what does not work (and is probably harmful) are low empathy and poor alliances. Paucity of support, collaboration, and consensus (as experienced by the client) predict treatment dropout and failure. The ineffective practitioner will also likely be incongruent in word and deed, be inclined to overlook alliance ruptures, and disregard emotional expression.

Another means of identifying relational elements that exert a negative influence is to scour research studies in search of those frequently associated with negative outcomes and premature discontinuation (e.g., Hardy et al.,

TABLE 5.1. Summary of Ineffective or Harmful Therapist Relational Behaviors

Ineffective	Harmful
Low empathy	Rigidity
Low collaboration	Confrontational style
Low consensus	Overconfidence
High reliance on therapist assessment of the alliance	Blame, criticism, hostility

2019; Swift & Greenberg, 2012). Harmful therapist behaviors include rigidity, overconfidence, and hostility. Confrontational style, criticism, rigidity, cultural arrogance (see Chapter 3), assumptions, and therapist-centricity (see Chapter 4) are also implicated (Norcross & Lambert, 2019; Soto et al., 2019). Because these behaviors and attitudes exert a potent negative impact, it makes sense from a DP perspective first to identify and mitigate their influence before turning attention to effective relationship factors.

As an example of rigidity, consider widespread policies mandating the use of specific treatment protocols and continued emphasis on training therapists in manualized treatments to the exclusion of relationship factors. Research shows neither adherence nor compliance with treatment manuals consistently relates to positive treatment outcomes (Collyer et al., 2020; Webb et al., 2010). More, strict adherence can cause a practitioner to overlook important client or relationship events, within and without of the therapy.

Statements of blame, sarcasm, criticism, or other hostility toward the client also powerfully predict poor outcome, with process studies indicating it does not require much animus in an otherwise typical session to create problems (Binder & Strupp, 1997). To be sure, readers of *Better Results* (*BR*; S. D. Miller et al., 2020) and the *FG* are unlikely to practice with an intentionally uncaring or critical style. Unfortunately, these relational behaviors can occur without therapist awareness. Research shows, for example, therapist assumptions about clients' experiences in therapy often don't align with the clients' actual experiences. While it might be tempting to believe clinicians can or should know—either by intuition or experience—when things are going well or badly with the relationship, studies clearly demonstrate it is not the case (Lambert, 2010); the client's perspective is more strongly related to outcome. In fact, meta-analytic research repeatedly advises therapists to privilege their clients' experience of the alliance, empathy, and outcome over their own (Norcross & Lambert, 2019).

Like other blind spots in human cognition, the conditions that promote these ineffective relational behaviors are often present in the environment and thus easily ignored. Insurance demands, practitioner anxiety, and external pressure to adhere to specific treatment techniques can create alliance-ruining rigidity. Frustration, defensiveness, fatigue, or inattentiveness can prompt hostile statements that practitioners might not even notice. The mere status of "health care expert" may compound the risk of making incorrect assumptions, engaging in dominant behavior, and being blind to cultural differences. Here, in particular, is where routinely soliciting feedback from clients, as described in *BR*, can prove critical, both in improving therapist responsiveness in the moment to the individual client, as well as identifying, via the aggregation of performance data, patterns of problematic relational behavior to target with DP.

Relationship Factors That Do Make a Difference

The empirical foundation on which this chapter rests is both mature and robust. Relationship factors all have effect sizes indicative of small to moderate benefit. Table 5.2 summarizes the results of meta-analyses. As can be seen,

TABLE 5.2. Summary of Meta-Analytic Results on Relationship Factors in Individual Psychotherapy

Relationship factor	# of studies *k*	# of patients *N*	Effect size *r*	*d* or *g*	Principle #
Empathy	82	6,138	.28	.58	3
Positive regard/affirmation	64	3,528	.28	.57	1
Congruence/genuineness	21	1,192	.23	.46	2
Real relationship	17	1,502	.37	.80	2
Emotional expression	42	925	.40	.85	4
Alliance (adult patients)	306	30,000+	.28	.57	3
Alliance (child & adolescent patients)	43	3,447	.20	.40	3
Collaboration	53	5,286	.29	.61	4
Goal consensus	54	7,278	.24	.49	3
Repairing alliance ruptures	11	1,318	.30	.62	1

Note. Adapted from "What Works in the Psychotherapy Relationship: Results, Conclusions, and Practices," by J. C. Norcross and M. J. Lambert, in J. C. Norcross and M. J. Lambert (Eds.), *Psychotherapy relationships that work* (3rd ed., Vol. 1, p. 367), 2019 (https://doi.org/10.1093/med-psych/9780190843953.001.0001). Copyright 2019 by J. C. Norcross and M. J. Lambert. Adapted with permission.

all nine of the factors listed have been designated effective. In short, no question, they all work (Norcross & Lambert, 2019).

In the material that follows, the evidence-based relationship factors are organized into two sets based roughly on their historical roots and groupings on the Taxonomy of Deliberate Practice Activities in Psychotherapy (TDPA; Chow & Miller, 2022; see Appendix A, this volume). The first set originated in the humanistic, client-centered literature and corresponds with TDPA Domain 3 (relationship), Subgroup B (Impact). The second set originated in the psychodynamic literature and corresponds with TDPA Domain 3 (relationship), Subgroupings A (effective focus) and D (difficulties).

Empathy

The term *empathy* is widely used to mean an array of experiences and behaviors that are *not* therapeutic empathy, such as a sympathetic response to the distress of another or recognizing superficial similarities between one's own experience and those of others. Such responses are self rather than client centered in nature (W. R. Miller, 2018). Therapeutic empathy occurs when the clinician seeks and then relays an accurate understanding of the client's feelings, perspectives, and experiences, as separate as possible from the therapist's own. In sum, an empathic stance is an antidote to the assumptions and therapist-centricity that prove ineffective for the therapy relationship.

Empathic responding is one of the strongest and best-supported contributors to outcome (Elliott et al., 2019). Starting with the groundbreaking research of Carl Rogers, decades of evidence now back up its value, with effect sizes ranging moderate to large ($d = .58$), from a whopping 82 high-quality studies. Even better, the skills and basic stance of empathic understanding can be practiced in everyday relationships outside of a real or simulated therapy situation (see W. R. Miller, 2018), as long as others in these relationships are willing and able to provide feedback. Such accessibility, paired with the strength of empathy's impact, makes it both one of the simplest and most ideal to translate into DP activities.

The meta-analytic research points to several central features of effective empathic responding (Elliott et al., 2019):

- Communication of attunement to the client's emotions and experiences. A narrow focus on the words the client says, or other concrete aspects of content, is not effective attunement, and neither is merely repeating back their words.

- Being flexible and open to new input from the client. Firm expectations or assumptions about the client should give way to attending and adjusting to clients' in-the-moment experience.

- Humility. Empathic listening involves educated guessing, stated as hypotheses with minimal assumptions. Trying to predict client views of their experiences (anticipatory empathy) is not particularly helpful.

FIELD GUIDE TIP

Chapter 8 of *BR* describes and illustrates how to mine your performance data for DP opportunities.

In light of the research on empathy presented in this section, consider sorting your clients based on their Session Rating Scale (or whatever relationship measure you are using) scores (good = 39–40, fair = 37–38, and poor 36 or lower), paying particular attention to the relation between the scores on the individual items, dropouts, and poor outcomes.

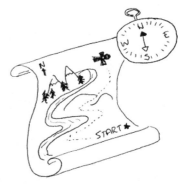

Positive Regard and Affirmation

Therapist positive regard for the client (and expression of that regard, including through affirmation) is another relationship factor originally investigated by Carl Rogers. As with empathy, positive regard has been the subject of much research since the early days of the field, with effect sizes falling in the moderate range ($d = .57$), based on 64 studies of quality appropriate for inclusion in a meta-analysis (Farber et al., 2019).

Like empathy, the terms *positive regard* and *affirmation* are easily misunderstood—mistaken for simple compliments, shallow praise, or other concrete tactics (e.g., preceding requests for compliance). In fact, positive regard is the therapist's genuine nonpossessive liking and expressed appreciation for the client as a unique person. Doing so strengthens the client's sense of agency and self. It is important to note that to contribute to outcome, this regard must be made evident to the client through words and nonverbal signals. Therapists can express on a regular basis, for example, in both verbal and nonverbal ways, that they value, care about, and believe in the client. Ideally, the therapist will experience and express such regard over the course of treatment. However, it does *not* need to be (and probably could not be) experienced by the therapist at every moment across treatment with any given client. Rogers made clear that positive regard should not be viewed as a stable characteristic of the relationship with a client (Farber et al., 2019).

Therapist Congruence/Genuineness and Real Relationship

This closely related pair of relational factors includes the last of the three classic Rogerian core conditions (empathy, unconditional positive regard, *and* congruence/genuineness) and a concept from the psychodynamic literature, the real relationship. Both have accumulated sufficient evidence to be classified as effective.

Congruence/genuineness has both intrapersonal and interpersonal features, meaning it is both a personal characteristic of the therapist as well as a quality of the therapeutic interaction. When congruent, therapists' actions and behaviors not only fit their words but also who they are as a person—their values and identity—exuding groundedness, thoughtfulness, and genuineness. In short, they are real, not phony, distracted, or playing a role. Studies of the factor show a moderate effect size, making it a reliable contributor to therapeutic success ($d = .46$; Kolden et al., 2019).

The real relationship is composed of both genuineness and realism. Gelso (2014) described it as "the personal relationship between therapist and patient marked by the extent to which each is genuine with the other and perceives/experiences the other in ways that befit the other" (p. 119). In contrast to the alliance, it refers to a subset of therapist–client interactions not directly focused on the tasks (Gelso et al., 2019). These interactions are taken at face value in the here and now. A meta-analysis based on 17 studies and 1,502 patients revealed a large effect between the real relationship and client success ($d = .80$; Gelso et al., 2019).

Emotional Expression

Although emotion is obviously core to psychotherapy, organized research on the subject is quite recent. Regardless, the evidence shows that the facilitation, experience, and expression of client emotion in session are strongly correlated with treatment outcome ($d = .85$; Peluso & Freund, 2019). Contributions to this research base come from a wider range of theoretical orientations than the factors reviewed thus far. Because of this variability, the definition of emotional expression is less precise and has failed to achieve consensus in the field. One essential and simple clarification: What is not being referenced here is the "expressed emotion" (EE) from family process and relapse prevention research with serious mental illnesses, where reducing EE is the goal. Consistent with the TDPA descriptions, the focus here is on therapist relational actions that facilitate client emotional expression in individual therapy (see TDPA Domain 3, Items Bi–v).

Of all the relational elements listed in the TDPA impact factor group (3B), emotional expression is possibly the most theory bound. It is also the one that can most clearly go astray in the absence of a clear plan. Treatment model and case formulation help determine which emotions to address, where a particular emotional expression fits into the therapeutic endeavor, and what to do with it—how to attend to and make therapeutic use of it versus allowing the session to deteriorate into an unfocused rant, wallow, panic, or self-attack.

Alliance in Adult Psychotherapy

The term *alliance* can be difficult to define and is not easily differentiated from several other relational concepts. Meaning varies depending on the theoretical orientation of the person using the term. In the professional literature, the words *working*, *helping*, or *therapeutic* often appear in conjunction with the term (Flückiger et al., 2019). An early tripartite definition by Bordin (1979) emphasized (a) a warm emotional bond, (b) agreement on respective tasks, and (c) consensus on treatment goals. A more recent definition includes mutual collaboration between client and therapist on goals and tasks of psychotherapy, along with the therapeutic bond between the dyad (Del Re et al., 2021). Because of the emphasis placed on mutual agreement and goal-directed movement, the alliance is difficult to assess without collecting information from, at minimum, the therapist and client.

At this point, a huge number of studies have been conducted on the relation of the alliance to client success. Across raters, a meta-analysis of more than 30,000 clients found a moderate but extremely robust association between the alliance and outcome in adult individual psychotherapy ($d = .57$; Flückiger et al., 2019). No doubt. The alliance relates, predicts, and contributes to success.

Alliance in Youth Psychotherapy

The therapeutic alliance also captures essential aspects of the relationship with children and adolescents. That said, proper measurement from the youth's perspective has been less common, and it is not clear whether youth collaboration on treatment goals is as central to the alliance as it is with adults (Karver et al., 2019). Nonetheless, it is important for the outcome of individual therapy that a child or adolescent experiences a warm bond with the therapist in a relationship focused on improving the young person's psychological functioning. The need to establish an alliance with a parent or caregiver when working with minors further complicates the picture. Such research and clinical challenges notwithstanding, a fair bit of evidence has accumulated. Across 43 studies of child and adolescent therapy (3,447 clients and parents), there is a moderate effect size between alliance and treatment outcome ($d = .40$; Karver et al., 2019). Importantly, the strength of alliance–outcome relation did not vary with the type of treatment. Further, the effect size, or clinical impact, of dual alliances—therapist with youth, therapist with parent—was identical. Bottom line: Both mightily matter.

Goal Consensus and Collaboration

These two factors are present across theoretical orientations and are sometimes considered part of the therapeutic alliance. Indeed, both are commonly assessed for research purposes via measures of the alliance, completed separately by clinician and client. Goal consensus refers to the agreement between the therapist and client about the targets of their work together and how to achieve them. Clarity of communication about treatment goals, degree of dedication to the endeavor, and a mutual understanding of how change will come about are also vital parts of that consensus. A large body of research documents the vital role this factor plays in outcome ($d = .49$; Tryon et al., 2019).

Collaboration is the active mutual engagement of the therapist and client around the work of therapy. Historically measured with subscales of alliance measures, recent studies of cognitive and behavioral therapies have conflated collaboration with completion of homework assignments. Simply put, while work between client and therapist often extends beyond the therapy hour, compliance is not collaboration. Research shows a substantial effect size for the latter ($d = .61$; Tryon et al., 2019).

Repairing Alliance Ruptures

Ruptures are problems or strains in the collaborative relationship between client and therapist (Safran et al., 2011) related to treatment goals, agreement on the tasks of therapy, or the emotional aspect of the dyad's collaborative bond (Eubanks et al., 2019). Two main types occur in session: (a) withdrawal, in which the client moves away from the therapist and the work, and (b) confrontation in which the client moves against the therapist, by expressing anger or dissatisfaction. Although the term *rupture* may connote a dramatic breakdown, many studies point to subtle tensions and minor misalignments as markers.

Therapist efforts to repair alliance ruptures can be overt or indirect. Either way, research shows attending to them improves treatment outcomes. A meta-analysis of 11 studies involving 1,318 clients revealed that repair of alliance ruptures in individual therapy is moderately to strongly associated with outcome ($d = .62$). That is, addressing ruptures works; ignoring them does not. Turns out, repairing ruptures is valuable for all therapists but is especially important for therapists with less experience and training in negotiating the therapeutic alliance (Eubanks et al., 2019). For example, a highly specialized statistical process known as moderator analysis reveals that rupture resolutions and training are particularly important for cognitive behavioral therapists, many of whom have not received explicit training in processing relationship dynamics with their clients.

EVIDENCE-BASED PRINCIPLES RELATED TO RELATIONSHIP FACTORS

Principle 1: Avoid the Don'ts, and When You (Invariably) Commit Them, Repair the Relationship

If the Golden Rule—a maxim found in most religions and cultures—constitutes sound advice for relationships in life, it can be considered an imperative in psychotherapy. Like the dos and don'ts reviewed in this chapter, the adage typically comes in one of two forms: positive ("Treat others as you would like others to treat you") and negative ("Do not treat others in ways that you would not like to be treated"). Flexibility, openness, and humility are research-supported examples of the former, as are being regularly affirming and providing positive regard. By contrast, who enjoys confrontation, being blamed or criticized, or met with sarcasm, arrogance, and rigidity? When ruptures occur, quickly repair them and fix the relationship.

Principle 2: Engage Genuinely in a Real Relationship

That all practitioners experience days where they are merely going through the motions, playing a role, or "phoning it in" is understandable. After all, conducting psychotherapy is ofttimes emotionally demanding and interpersonally grueling work. Of all the relationship factors, engaging in a real relationship—composed of genuineness and realism—is among the most potent. Mindful self-awareness is key, including being accepting of self, behaving responsively to the client, and manifesting both intrapersonal and interpersonal congruence.

Principle 3: Attune, Align, and Collaborate for Impact

For both young and old, it is the client's experience of the therapist and the treatment that matters *most*. The essential questions are the following: Do *they* feel heard and understood? Is the therapist empathically attuned to *their* inner experience? Do *they* feel supported and validated? Is *their* relationship with the therapist collaborative in nature and aligned with *their* goals? Better results are achieved when the answers to the foregoing questions are in the affirmative.

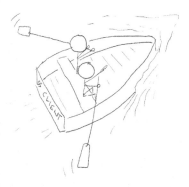

Principle 4: Facilitate Emotional Expression and Processing for Best Results

It is self-evident that clients have feelings, but for decades, most practitioners did not know what to do with them except to listen. New psychotherapy research and affective neuroscience converge in directing practitioners to help clients experience, express, and process those emotions. That leads to more client health and happiness. The best results ensue when therapists process feelings consistent with a treatment model and case formulation.

EXERCISES FOR RELATIONSHIP FACTOR SKILL DEVELOPMENT

To be effective, the DP exercises you choose must help you reach for performance objectives just beyond your current abilities. As such, prior to reviewing the following exercises, ensure you have taken all of the steps outlined in the decision tree presented at the start of this chapter. It is assumed you have (a) routinely measured your performance, (b) collected sufficient data to establish a reliable profile of your therapeutic effectiveness, (c) completed the TDPA, (d) determined a deficit exists in your performance related to relationship factors, (e) narrowed your focus to a single element within the relationship factors domain on the TDPA, and (f) defined that performance improvement objective in SMART terms (specific, measurable, achievable, relevant, and time bound). Next, choose an exercise that aligns most closely with your goal. Remember, "deliberate practice is a marathon, not a sprint" (S. D. Miller et al., 2020, p. 58). Pacing and planning are essential for sustaining the effort necessary for success. Should none of the exercises speak directly to your needs, Chapter 2 can provide guidance for developing your own.

Exercise 1: Buddy Up for Improvement

Principle: 1
Applicability: TDPA Items 3Aiii, iv, 3Bi–iv, 3Di, iv
Purpose
Personal soul-searching—even reviewing recordings of our own work—may not reveal our subtle rigidity and negative process (e.g., negativity, hostility, sarcasm) in session. Supervision, third-party observation, and feedback from clients offer the possibility of a broader perspective.

Task
Together with your clinical supervisor or colleague, watch recordings of three sessions with different clients. Optimize your selection by choosing sessions (a) that have ended with low scores on whatever alliance/relationship scale you administer (e.g., Session Rating Scale [SRS]), (b) that have been followed by the client dropping out of treatment, or (c) during which you experienced negative emotions toward the client.

   DP must be cognitively taxing to be effective, so start by dedicating a half hour to the process described next. Begin by watching a video, stopping at points where more flexible/responsive, less critical/hostile responses were possible but missed. With the help of your colleague or supervisor, craft at least two alternative responses. For each of these, imagine what a client might say and how you would respond in an open and empathic manner.

For this exercise to be useful, commit to reviewing videos in this way at least once a week for a month or more. Be forewarned: Watching our mistakes on video in front of peers can prove ego bruising, but it is the courageous way forward to better treatment results. As your comfort level increases, ask your supervisor or peer to role-play more challenging reactions to the alternative responses you craft. Note if and how your good partnership "do's" are improving over time.

Exercise 2: Back to the Classic

Principle: 3
Applicability: TDPA Item 3Bi, v (also applicable to 4C, E)
Purpose
The quality of a therapist's empathic attunement cannot be accurately assessed via intuition or deep reflection. We simply are not in possession of the client's perception without systematically welcoming and obtaining it.

Task
Write the names of your active clients on separate slips of paper. When done, mix all the names together in a hat (or box). For the first 15 slips drawn, begin administering the classic Barrett-Lennard Relationship Inventory (from Barrett-Lennard, 2015, or online at various sites). After calculating the range (i.e., highest and lowest) and average of your clients' scores,

- compare each client's score from session to session, considering what contributed to increases or decreases.

- compare your average score with that of the normative sample, reflecting on how your clients typically experience your empathic attunement. Look specifically at those clients whose scores fall below the norms.

- identify any cases of declining scores (while being mindful of research reviewed earlier in this chapter showing empathic attunement is associated with better outcomes). Use the method described in Exercise 1 (Buddying Up for Improvement) to foster the development of more helpful alternatives.

- from month to month, repeat the exercise as described. As data accumulate, sort the scores by age, gender identity, diagnosis, or culture, identifying any groupings where you perform more poorly on the Barrett-Lennard Relationship Inventory. Empathic responding includes sensitivity and adjustment to the individual client and the singular moment. That includes attending and responding therapeutically to those for whom conventional, Rogerian empathic responses do not prove ideal, as well as clients with whom—consciously or unconsciously—you offer suboptimal understanding.

- use the method described in Exercise 1 (Buddying Up for Improvement) to foster the development of more helpful alternatives.

Remember, even if unpleasant in the beginning, the data are always friendly in the long run. If the results are supportive of your perceived empathic quality with most clients, then, by all means, move on to remediating other relational skills. If the results are not supportive, devoting additional time to enhancing your empathic skills can definitely make a difference in your clinical results.

Exercise 3: Only Connect (E. M. Forster, *Howards End*)

Principle: 3
Applicability: TDPA Item 3Bi, v (also applicable to 4C, D, E; 5Aiv, viii, 5Bi)
Purpose
According to research reviews, the best skill training in empathy begins with didactics and ends with experiential elements (Elliott et al., 2019). This exercise joins these two critical elements using William R. Miller's (2018) book *Listening Well: The Art of Empathic Understanding.* As you will see, this slim volume contains didactics presented in brief, clear sections and supported by numerous exercises designed to improve skills for warm, accurate listening to another person. The exercises can be done in any reasonably close relationship, providing plenty of opportunities for practice and refinement of skills outside of therapy.

Task
On pages 14–18, W. R. Miller provides a real gem, a list of 12 roadblocks to empathic listening. These will surprise many people because they include an array of behaviors that are commonly employed in what are believed to be "positive" conversations in daily life (e.g., probing, agreeing, reassuring) but that interfere with true empathic listening. Instead of helping clients develop a deeper understanding of what they are feeling and what they mean to say, these behaviors stop them in their tracks.

Begin by printing the list of the 12 roadblocks and keeping them handy. Then, for a month, whenever an opportunity presents for a conversation with a colleague or friend, ask if they would help you with a brief experiment. Let them know nothing special is required on their part. The two of you will talk briefly, and you will ask for feedback about the experience. Should they agree, continue the conversation, interjecting as many of the roadblock responses as possible in the first 5 minutes. Each should be short and sweet, taking advantage of whatever opportunity naturally arises in the conversation—for example, judging ("You should really do that. You need to . . .") and agreeing ("Yes, yes, you're right"). Using a scale from 1 to 10, ask the listener to rate how well they felt heard and understood. For the next 5 minutes, avoid as many of the roadblocks as you can. It will prove more difficult than you probably imagine. Once again, ask the person to rate their experience of being heard and understood. Keep notes about your experience and learnings.

Return to *Listening Well* and pay particular attention to Chapter 8, Forming Reflections. Here you will find specific instructions and examples for developing the positive behaviors that, used in combination with real attention to the speaker (instead of divided attention while thinking of what to say next or what you want them to do), will foster better empathic understanding. Here's a warning and some advice: The exercise W. R. Miller suggests appears so simple you might think you already do it well. Practice it with one or two of your close friends, and you will soon discover it is far more challenging.

Begin by soliciting a commitment from a friend or colleague to help you practice your listening skills. Ten to 15 minutes is all that is required, with meetings spread out over an extended period of time (e.g., 1 month), thereby leaving time in between for reflection and consolidation of learning. Begin each meeting by having the person say, "Something you should know about me is that I am _____," ending with an adjective that is open to interpretation. Follow their statement with a reflection, which will be your best guess or hypothesis about the feeling, motivation, or value contained in what the speaker said. Importantly, your response must *not* be stated as a question and should end with downward voice intonation. The speaker follows, either letting you know you are right or wrong or clarifying. Based on their reply, you offer another reflection, the process continuing through several turns in conversation. The challenge for the listener is remembering to reflect not only the original statement but also the new information added at each turn. At the end of the conversation, ask for detailed feedback from your friend/listener, noting, in particular, those times when they felt you had truly heard what they were attempting to communicate. Note that most find achieving consistency in their reflections difficult! Be patient. Keep a log of your learnings.

Exercise 4: What Would Carl Rogers Do?

Principle: 2, 3
Applicability: TDPA Item 3Bi, ii (also applicable to 4D, 5Aii)
Purpose
Rarely do we recommend reading or watching recordings as efficacious methods of DP. The one exception is the work of Carl Ransom Rogers. His published writings and video demonstrations (beyond the infamous *Gloria* or *Three Approaches to Psychotherapy*) on the core facilitative conditions of psychotherapy should be a part of every health care practitioner's professional development, particularly on the subject of unconditional positive regard.

Task
Part 1. Decide to immerse yourself in Rogers's work, locating articles, books, and recordings. Over the course of a month or more, for no more than an hour at a time, study his writings or watch videos. Absorb the complexity and variety of how he talks about and expresses unconditional regard. Pay particular attention to how he exudes it in so many ways. Be patient. It's likely to take time. As he observed, "Tis a way of being" (Rogers, 1980), not a technique.

Using pen and paper or using your favorite note-keeping app, keep a log of your observations and learnings, paying particular attention to the "sweet spots" in what he did and said. When watching a video of him working with a client, use the stop–start technique—specifically, stopping the recording *prior* to Rogers's turn in conversation, first writing down how you would respond and then comparing it with what he said. Keep in mind your reflections about the difference are more important than getting the wording exactly right. You will know you are making progress when you (a) jettison the common yet antiquated notion that Rogers simply fed clients compliments, (b) accumulate new ways of communicating positive regard, and (c) spontaneously find yourself experiencing more genuine nonpossessive liking of and appreciation for your clients' uniqueness.

Part 2. Part 2 of this exercise might be called "Walk in Your Client's Shoes." The expression is being used here literally rather than figuratively. Part of communicating respect and care for the people we work with is creating a safe, peaceful, and nourishing physical environment. Begin by reflecting on your "therapy space": the communications clients have prior to their first appointment, where they enter the building, your waiting area, and your consulting room (even if online). Consider the ambience, color, sound, lighting, safety, ventilation, flooring, and furniture. Are the reading materials in the waiting room organized, clean, and current? Are the chairs comfortable? Is the artwork meaningful? What is the overall feeling? End by asking five nontherapists to visit. While you wait outside, have them sit in your waiting area and office, noting their immediate impressions. Embrace any discrepancies as feedback.

Other environmental features to consider? Paperwork, billing, and any measures you typically ask clients to complete. Evaluate what these procedures and experiences communicate. Do they adequately convey positive regard—an appreciation of the uniqueness of each individual client? Once again, walk five nontherapists through your process. Ask them to reflect on the experience, noting what feelings it conjures or inspires. Consider creating a learning project, as described in Chapters 2 and 9, aimed at rectifying what is unsatisfactory in the environment you seek to project. Make small tweaks and then repeat the exercise every 6 months to ensure your therapy environment represents the best of you.

Exercise 5: Set Your Heart Right (Confucius)

Principle: 2
Applicability: TDPA Item 3Biii, iv (also applicable to 5Avi)
Purpose
Congruence is both intrapersonal (therapist quality) and interpersonal (relational) in nature. Mindfulness, stretching, and relaxation may all help in "setting your heart right" for meeting with clients. Indeed, a multisite randomized controlled trial found that therapists who practiced presession mindfulness were more present in their meetings with clients. However, it did not necessarily

result in them becoming more effective (Dunn et al., 2013). While disappointing, such a finding will *not* come as a surprise to anyone who understands DP. As noted in Chapter 1, to be effective, the time you devote to professional development must be aimed at helping you reach for objectives just beyond your current ability. The process begins by using data to identify performance deficits.

Task

At the end of each day spent meeting with clients, take a few moments to review those sessions where you experienced a lack of congruence either internally or in the therapeutic interaction. In 100 words or less, write down the client and time of day and any other factors you consider contributary. After you have completed the process a minimum 10 times, retrieve your notes, sorting the collection into themes. Refine the list by continuing the exercise additional days.

Develop a plan for addressing the dominant themes (e.g., engaging in presession mindfulness practices, decreasing the number of clients seen or the times of day you meet clients, committing to leaving enough time between visits to read through case notes prior to meeting). Review your plans with a trusted colleague, supervisor, or expert consultant.

Exercise 6: Go to the Tape

Principle: 4
Applicability: TDPA Items 3Bii, iii, vi, 3Dii, iii, iv (also applicable to 1K, 5Ai,ii)
Purpose
Psychotherapy sessions are often affective crucibles in which neither patient nor practitioner recall proves accurate about the expression and processing of in-session emotion. Thus, observer ratings may be better sources of information than either therapist or client postsession report in determining when the therapist unintentionally dampens the experience and expression of emotion.

Task

Part 1. If you have not already started doing so, begin recording your work (with informed consent, of course). Identify those sessions in which the client expressed a meager amount of emotion. Next, block out 30 minutes of uninterrupted time. For the first 20, watch one of the recordings. Beware! Audio and video are dense mediums. To guard against information overload, limit your focus to a single objective: finding exchanges during the hour in which your verbal response (or lack thereof) unintentionally dampened the client's experience, expression, or processing of emotions. Think of this exercise as a fine-grained analysis of response couplets that did not lead to or result in affective experiencing in places that the research evidence and your treatment model would deem desirable.

After locating at least four exchanges, spend the last 10 minutes reflecting on the reasons (both conscious and partly unconscious) for your discouraging or minimizing client emotions. Does it feel too painful? Are you uncomfortable with strong affect? Are you too fatigued to take it on? Are there any patterns to your behavior? What might a different response look like that feels congruent to you and your therapeutic approach?

Part 2. Early on in *BR,* you were asked to create a schematic or blueprint for how you do therapy sufficiently detailed so another practitioner could understand and replicate it—literally, "step into your shoes" and work how you work (S. D. Miller et al., 2020, p. 29). The purpose of the exercise was to make it possible for clinicians to pinpoint where they could intervene once data-derived performance improvement opportunities were identified. In response to reader feedback, a more detailed description (and hopefully improved) version was developed and included in the *FG* (see pp. 18–20, Chapter 1). If you have not completed the activity, please do so now.

Next, with your completed "map" in hand, consider where, when, and how client emotional expression plays a part in your treatment approach. If it is *not* mentioned explicitly, add it, taking time to identify how it is related to your theoretical premises and overall plan of action. Finish this activity by returning to the exchanges from the recording you reviewed and, for each, writing out how specifically you would invite client emotional experiencing and expression consistent with your therapeutic approach. Wait to check for progress until you have repeated the exercise a couple of times per week for at least a month. You can do so by reviewing recordings of subsequent sessions with the same clients.

Exercise 7: Rate and Predict

Principle: 3
Applicability: TDPA Items 3Ai–iv, 3Cii, vi (also applicable to 1D-F, 4A, B, E)
Purpose
The good news is training in alliance building frequently results in improved therapeutic alliances in session; the bad news is such training takes a fair bit of practitioner time and effort (e.g., Ackerman & Hilsenroth, 2003; Crits-Christoph et al., 2006; Muran et al., 2018). As *alignment* with another literally means being in a state of agreeing or matching, success requires knowing when a difference between our clients and us exists. This activity is designed to foster such awareness.

Task
At the end of each session, while your clients complete the SRS, fill one out yourself from the client's perspective. The aim is to be altered or disconfirmed, not confirmed. Why? As noted in Chapter 1, our brains are hardwired for novelty. Simply put, we listen better when we confront challenging or surprising situations. Continue the activity for a month, keeping notes about what you

learn. Once again, sort for patterns. Are there certain clients, presenting problems, times of day, or days of the week when you are more likely to be misaligned?

Exercise 8: I Am Clueless

Principle: 3
Applicability: TDPA Items 3Ai, ii (also applicable to 1F, H, I, 2B, 4A, B, E)
Purpose
Treatment planning and the popularity of so-called SMART goals can inadvertently lead to viewing therapeutic objectives as static in nature. In truth, the goals, meaning, or purpose of treatment are constantly evolving. At best, goals should be viewed as temporary signposts—verbs rather than nouns—subject to change as progress is achieved (or not) over an episode of care. The purpose of this exercise is twofold: (a) improve therapist awareness of and adjustment to client goals, and (b) increase therapist awareness and integration of other stakeholders' concerns, hopes, and objectives.

Task
Randomly select 10 clients from your caseload with whom you have met at least twice but no more than five times. In advance of your next scheduled visit, write what you believe their goals to be. Note if their goals have evolved since the start of treatment. When you next meet, ask those clients something along the following lines: "Let's take a moment and check back in on what you hope to accomplish here. Pretend I am clueless about your goals for psychotherapy. What would you say they are?" Continue the process for several weeks or until you have collected data from 30 total clients. Once done, begin systematically comparing their answers with your own written answers, noting the level of agreement and degree of divergence. What patterns, if any, emerge? Consider the level and rate in your work with mandated clients, youth, couples,

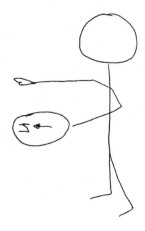

FIELD GUIDE TIP

For the cases you review in Exercise 8, retrieve each client's completed Session Rating Scale. Note whether any identified misalignment regarding the client's goals and objectives is reflected in lower scores on the second item on the measure. If not, consider how you might prompt the client to provide more accurate in-session feedback (see TDPA Items 1iii–vi).

or families. Is it more or less frequent? Should discrepancies be apparent, keep a log of who you tend to align with more and less often. Sort for patterns, eventually devoting time to developing a plan for improving collaboration and consensus addressing the dominant themes (e.g., engagement in presession mindfulness practices, decreasing the number of clients seen or the times of day you meet clients, committing to leaving enough time between visits to read through case notes prior to meeting). Review your ideas with a trusted colleague, supervisor, or expert consultant.

Exercise 9: Repairing Ruptures

Principle: 1
Applicability: TDPA Items 3Bii, Di (also applicable to 5Ai, ii, iv)
Purpose
When it comes to alliance ruptures in psychotherapy, repairing is literally about re-pairing the therapist with the client. No exact prescription for handling ruptures exists. Equipping therapists with the skills necessary to derive their own personalized solutions (Eubanks et al., 2019) entails

- recognizing ruptures when they occur (both withdrawal and confrontation ruptures),
- tolerating the difficult emotions they evoke,
- affirming clients for expressing their discontent (even if indirectly), and
- responding in empathic and flexible ways.

Task
Part 1. If you have identified rupture repair as a target for DP—either because of specific metrics in your performance data (e.g., high dropout rate, low SRS scores, or client report) or because of completion of the TDPA—your first step is to reflect on your history. Of the four skills listed earlier, note which, whether in your clinical work or personal therapy, proves the most challenging. After doing so, create a learning project. Read. Watch and/or engage an expert. Role-play outside the session—again, reenacting clients or therapists you have met.

Part 2. Start by making a "collection basket." When you experience a rupture with a client or hear one reported by a colleague, write it down and add it to your collection. Once you have 10 or more, pick two confrontation ruptures (e.g., an adolescent complaining that "you always take my parents' side"; an older client responding to your well-intended expression of understanding with "You still don't get me at all") and two withdrawal ruptures (e.g., a child physically and verbally withdrawing from the session, an adult manifesting standoffish discontent but not verbalizing it). Next, record family members or friends briefly reenacting the ruptures. Play the recording and write out a response, mindful of incorporating the four skills noted earlier. Continue the exercise until the scenarios have been exhausted.

FURTHER READING AND RESOURCES

This chapter reviewed the research evidence, identified evidence-based principles, and suggested DP exercises for working with relationship factors in psychotherapy. Additional research and recommendations can be found in the following:

- Two well-validated and clinically relevant measures for assessing and improving relationship skills are (a) Barrett-Lennard, G. T. (2015). *The Relationship Inventory: A complete resource and guide.* Wiley-Blackwell, and (b) Facilitative Interpersonal Skills inventory, available at https://www.fisresearch.com.

- Detailed review of the research and description of the real relationship and the therapeutic alliance can be found in Gelso, C. J. (2018). *The therapeutic relationship in psychotherapy practice: An integrative perspective.* Routledge.

- As noted in the body of the chapter, William R. Miller's (2018) *Listening Well: The Art of Empathic Understanding* is an excellent resource.

- A framework and detailed instructions for helping clients develop goals, including creating stakeholder awareness, can be found in classic articles by Karl Tomm: Tomm, K. (1987). Interventive interviewing: Part II. Reflexive Questioning as a means to enable self-healing. *Family Process, 26*(2), 167–183. https://doi.org/10.1111/j.1545-5300.1987.00167.x; Tomm, K. (1988). Interventive Interviewing: Part III: Intending to ask lineal, circular, strategic or reflexive questions. *Family Process, 27*(1), 1–15. https://doi.org/10.1111/j.1545-5300.1988.00001.x

- The Society for the Advancement of Psychotherapy (APA Division of Psychotherapy) has created videos and resources for learning and teaching relationship factors. They can be accessed free of cost at https://societyforpsychotherapy.org/teaching-learning-evidence-based-relationships/

- Practice recommendations and case examples specific to each of the reviewed relationship factors can be found in Norcross, J. C., & Lambert, M. J. (2019). (Eds.). *Psychotherapy relationships that work: Volume 1. Evidence-based therapist contributions* (3rd ed.). Oxford University Press.

- The research evidence on personalizing or adapting therapy to the individual client can be found in Norcross, J. C., & Wampold, B. E. (2019). (Eds.). *Psychotherapy relationships that work: Volume 2. Evidence-based responsiveness* (3rd ed.). Oxford University Press.

REFERENCES

Ackerman, S. J., & Hilsenroth, M. J. (2003). A review of therapist characteristics and techniques positively impacting the therapeutic alliance. *Clinical Psychology Review, 23*(1), 1–33. https://doi.org/10.1016/S0272-7358(02)00146-0

Anderson, T., Finkelstein, J. D., & Horvath, S. A. (2020). The facilitative interpersonal skills method: Difficult psychotherapy moments and appropriate therapist responsiveness. *Counselling and Psychotherapy Research, 20*(3), 463–469. https://doi.org/10.1002/capr.12302

Barrett-Lennard, G. T. (2015). *The Relationship Inventory: A complete resource and guide.* Wiley-Blackwell.

Binder, J. L., & Strupp, H. H. (1997). "Negative process": A recurrently discovered and underestimated facet of therapeutic process and outcome in the individual psychotherapy of adults. *Clinical Psychology: Science and Practice, 4*(2), 121–139. https://doi.org/10.1111/j.1468-2850.1997.tb00105.x

Bordin, E. S. (1979). The generalizability of the psychoanalytic concept of the working alliance. *Psychotherapy, 16*(3), 252–260. https://doi.org/10.1037/h0085885

Burlingame, G. M., McClendon, D. T., & Yang, C. (2019). Cohesion in group therapy. In J. C. Norcross & M. J. Lambert (Eds.), *Psychotherapy relationships that work* (3rd ed., Vol. 1, pp. 205–244). Oxford University Press. https://doi.org/10.1093/med-psych/9780190843953.003.0006

Castonguay, L. G., & Hill, C. E. (Eds.). (2017). *How and why are some therapists better than others? Understanding therapist effects.* American Psychological Association. https://doi.org/10.1037/0000034-000

Chow, D., & Miller, S. D. (2022). *Taxonomy of Deliberate Practice Activities in Psychotherapy—Therapist Version* (Version 6). International Center for Clinical Excellence.

Collyer, H., Eisler, I., & Woolgar, M. (2020). Systematic literature review and meta-analysis of the relationship between adherence, competence and outcome in psychotherapy for children and adolescents. *European Child & Adolescent Psychiatry, 29*(4), 417–431. https://doi.org/10.1007/s00787-018-1265-2

Crits-Christoph, P., Gibbons, M. B. C., Crits-Christoph, K., Narducci, J., Schamberger, M., & Gallop, R. (2006). Can therapists be trained to improve their alliances? A preliminary study of alliance-fostering psychotherapy. *Psychotherapy Research, 16*(3), 268–281. https://doi.org/10.1080/10503300500268557

Del Re, A. C., Flückiger, C., Horvath, A. O., & Wampold, B. E. (2021). Examining therapist effects in the alliance-outcome relationship: A multilevel meta-analysis. *Journal of Consulting and Clinical Psychology, 89*(5), 371–378. https://doi.org/10.1037/ccp0000637

Dunn, R., Callahan, J. L., Swift, J. K., & Ivanovic, M. (2013). Effects of pre-session centering for therapists on session presence and effectiveness. *Psychotherapy Research, 23*(1), 78–85. https://doi.org/10.1080/10503307.2012.731713

Elliott, R., Bohart, A. C., Watson, J. C., & Murphy, D. (2019). Empathy. In J. C. Norcross & M. J. Lambert (Eds.), *Psychotherapy relationships that work* (3rd ed., Vol. 1, pp. 245–287). Oxford University Press. https://doi.org/10.1093/med-psych/9780190843953.003.0007

Eubanks, C. F., Muran, J. C., & Safran, J. D. (2019). Repairing alliance ruptures. In J. C. Norcross & M. J. Lambert (Eds.), *Psychotherapy relationships that work* (3rd ed., Vol. 1, pp. 549–579). Oxford University Press. https://doi.org/10.1093/med-psych/9780190843953.003.0016

Farber, B. A., Suzuki, J. Y., & Lynch, D. (2019). Positive regard and affirmation. In J. C. Norcross & M. J. Lambert (Eds.), *Psychotherapy relationships that work* (3rd ed., Vol. 1, pp. 288–322). Oxford University Press. https://doi.org/10.1093/med-psych/9780190843953.003.0008

Flückiger, C., Del Re, A. C., Wampold, B. E., Symonds, D., & Horvath, A. O. (2019). Alliance in adult psychotherapy. In J. C. Norcross & M. J. Lambert (Eds.), *Psychotherapy relationships that work* (3rd ed., Vol. 1, pp. 24–78). Oxford University Press. https://doi.org/10.1093/med-psych/9780190843953.003.0002

Friedlander, M. L., Escudero, V., Welmers-van de Poll, M. J., & Heatherington, L. (2019). Alliances in couple and family therapy. In J. C. Norcross & M. J. Lambert (Eds.),

Psychotherapy relationships that work (3rd ed., Vol. 1, pp. 117–166). Oxford University Press. https://doi.org/10.1093/med-psych/9780190843953.003.0004

Gelso, C. (2014). A tripartite model of the therapeutic relationship: Theory, research, and practice. *Psychotherapy Research, 24*(2), 117–131. https://doi.org/10.1080/10503307.2013.845920

Gelso, C. J., & Carter, J. A. (1985). The relationship in counseling and psychotherapy: Components, consequences, and theoretical antecedents. *The Counseling Psychologist, 13*(2), 155–243. https://doi.org/10.1177/0011000085132001

Gelso, C. J., & Carter, J. A. (1994). Components of the psychotherapy relationship: Their inter-action and unfolding during treatment. *Journal of Counseling Psychology, 41*(3), 296–306. https://doi.org/10.1037/0022-0167.41.3.296

Gelso, C. J., Kivlighan, D. M., Jr., & Markin, R. D. (2019). The real relationship. In J. C. Norcross & M. J. Lambert (Eds.), *Psychotherapy relationships that work* (3rd ed., Vol. 1, pp. 351–378). Oxford University Press. https://doi.org/10.1093/med-psych/9780190843953.003.0010

Hardy, G. E., Bishop-Edwards, L., Chambers, E., Connell, J., Dent-Brown, K., Kothari, G., O'hara, R., & Parry, G. D. (2019). Risk factors for negative experiences during psycho-therapy. *Psychotherapy Research, 29*(3), 403–414. https://doi.org/10.1080/10503307.2017.1393575

Hendrix, H. (2007). *Getting the love you want: A guide for couples* (20th ed.). Macmillan.

Horvath, A. O., Symonds, D. B., Flückiger, C., DelRe, A. C., & Lee, E. (2016, June 16–18). Integration across professional domains: The helping relationship. In A. O. Horvath (Chair), *How do therapists contribute to positive outcomes? The opinions of three experienced psychologists* [Symposium]. Society for the Exploration of Psychotherapy Integration 32nd Annual Convention, Dublin, Ireland.

Karver, M. S., De Nadai, A. S., Monahan, M., & Shirk, S. R. (2019). Alliance in child and adolescent psychotherapy. In J. C. Norcross & M. J. Lambert (Eds.), *Psychotherapy relationships that work* (3rd ed., Vol. 1, pp. 79–116). Oxford University Press. https://doi.org/10.1093/med-psych/9780190843953.003.0003

Knox, S., & Hill, C. E. (2021). Training and supervision in psychotherapy: What we know and where we need to go. In M. Barkham, W. Lutz, & L. G. Castonguay (Eds.), *Bergin and Garfield's handbook of psychotherapy and behavior change* (7th ed., pp. 327–350). Wiley.

Kolden, G. G., Wang, C. C., Austin, S. B., Chang, Y., & Klein, M. H. (2019). Congruence/genuineness. In J. C. Norcross & M. J. Lambert (Eds.), *Psychotherapy relationships that work* (3rd ed., Vol. 1, pp. 323–350). Oxford University Press. https://doi.org/10.1093/med-psych/9780190843953.003.0009

Lambert, M. J. (2010). *Prevention of treatment failure: The use of measuring, monitoring, & feedback in clinical practice.* American Psychological Association. https://doi.org/10.1037/12141-000

Lambert, M. J., & Hill, C. E. (1994). Assessing psychotherapy outcomes and processes. In A. E. Bergin & S. L. Garfield (Eds.), *Handbook of psychotherapy and behavior change* (4th ed., pp. 72–113). Wiley.

Miller, S. D., Hubble, M. A., & Chow, D. (2020). *Better results: Using deliberate practice to improve therapeutic effectiveness.* American Psychological Association. https://doi.org/10.1037/0000191-000

Miller, W. R. (2018). *Listening well: The art of empathic understanding.* Wipf and Stock.

Miller, W. R., & Rollnick, S. (2012). *Motivational interviewing: Helping people change.* Guilford Press.

Muran, J. C., Safran, J. D., Eubanks, C. F., & Gorman, B. S. (2018). The effect of alliance-focused training on a cognitive-behavioral therapy for personality dis-orders. *Journal of Consulting and Clinical Psychology, 86*(4), 384–397. https://doi.org/10.1037/ccp0000284

Nienhuis, J. B., Owen, J., Valentine, J. C., Black, S. W., Halford, T. C., Parazak, S. E., Budge, S., & Hilsenroth, M. (2018). Therapeutic alliance, empathy, and genuineness in individual adult psychotherapy: A meta-analytic review. *Psychotherapy Research, 28*(4), 593–605. https://doi.org/10.1080/10503307.2016.1204023

Norcross, J. C., & Cooper, M. (2021). *Personalizing psychotherapy: Assessing and accommodating patient preferences*. American Psychological Association. https://doi.org/10.1037/0000221-000

Norcross, J. C., & Lambert, M. J. (Eds.). (2019). *Psychotherapy relationships that work* (3rd ed., Vol. 1). Oxford University Press. https://doi.org/10.1093/med-psych/9780190843953.001.0001

Norcross, J. C., & Wampold, B. E. (Eds.). (2019). *Psychotherapy relationships that work* (3rd ed., Vol. 2). Oxford University Press.

Orlinsky, D. E., Grawe, K., & Parks, B. K. (1994). Process and outcome in psychotherapy—Noch einmal. In A. E. Bergin & S. L. Garfield (Eds.), *Handbook of psychotherapy and behavior change* (4th ed., pp. 270–376). Wiley.

Peluso, P. R., & Freund, R. R. (2019). Emotional expression. In J. C. Norcross & M. J. Lambert (Eds.), *Psychotherapy relationships that work* (3rd ed., Vol. 1, pp. 421–460). Oxford University Press. https://doi.org/10.1093/med-psych/9780190843953.003.0012

Ripken, C. (2019). *Just show up and other enduring values from baseball's iron man*. HarperCollins.

Rogers, C. R. (1980). *A way of being*. Houghton Mifflin.

Safran, J. D., Muran, J. C., & Eubanks-Carter, C. (2011). Repairing alliance ruptures. *Psychotherapy, 48*(1), 80–87. https://doi.org/10.1037/a0022140

Soto, A., Smith, T. B., Griner, D., Rodriguez, M. D., & Bernal, G. (2019). Cultural adaptations and multicultural competence. In J. C. Norcross & B. E. Wampold (Eds.), *Psychotherapy relationships that work* (Vol. 2, pp. 86–132). Oxford University Press. https://doi.org/10.1093/med-psych/9780190843960.003.0004

Swift, J. K., & Greenberg, R. P. (2012). Premature discontinuation in adult psychotherapy: A meta-analysis. *Journal of Consulting and Clinical Psychology, 80*(4), 547–559. https://doi.org/10.1037/a0028226

Totura, C. M. W., Fields, S. A., & Karver, M. S. (2018). The role of the therapeutic relationship in psychopharmacological treatment outcomes: A meta-analytic review. *Psychiatric Services, 69*(1), 41–47. https://doi.org/10.1176/appi.ps.201700114

Tryon, G. S., Birch, S. E., & Verkuilen, J. (2019). Goal consensus and collaboration. In J. C. Norcross & M. J. Lambert (Eds.), *Psychotherapy relationships that work* (3rd ed., Vol. 1, pp. 167–204). Oxford University Press.

Wampold, B. E., & Imel, Z. (2015). *The great psychotherapy debate* (2nd ed.). Erlbaum. https://doi.org/10.4324/9780203582015

Watson, J. C., & Geller, S. (2005). An examination of the relations among empathy, unconditional acceptance, positive regard and congruence in both cognitive-behavioral and process-experiential psychotherapy. *Psychotherapy Research, 15*(1–2), 25–33. https://doi.org/10.1080/10503300512331327010

Webb, C. A., Derubeis, R. J., & Barber, J. P. (2010). Therapist adherence/competence and treatment outcome: A meta-analytic review. *Journal of Consulting and Clinical Psychology, 78*(2), 200–211. https://doi.org/10.1037/a0018912

Hope and Expectancy Factors

Michael J. Constantino, Heather J. Muir, Averi N. Gaines, and
Kimberly Ouimette

*Expectation colored by hope and faith is an effective force with which we have to reckon . . .
in all our attempts at treatment and cure.*

—SIGMUND FREUD, *THE COMPLETE PSYCHOLOGICAL
WORKS OF SIGMUND FREUD*

DECISION POINT

Begin here if you have read the book *Better Results* and

- are routinely measuring your performance *and*
- have collected sufficient data to establish a reliable, evidence-based profile
  of your therapeutic effectiveness *and*
- have completed the Taxonomy of Deliberate Practice Activities in
  Psychotherapy *and*
- need help developing deliberate practice exercises that leverage hope and
  expectancy factors.

In the celebration and discussion of methods and techniques, central elements
in successful therapy—hope and expectancy—more often than not receive
scant attention. This is unfortunate because current evidence convincingly
demonstrates these critical components have a significant influence at the

---

https://doi.org/10.1037/0000358-007
The Field Guide to Better Results: Evidence-Based Exercises to Improve Therapeutic Effectiveness,
S. D. Miller, D. Chow, S. Malins, and M. A. Hubble (Editors)

beginning and throughout the course of treatment, potentiating an eventual positive result. Furthermore, specific, trainable therapist skills exist that can cultivate clients' hope and expectancy, in any type of therapy, in a way that is helpful for both engagement (i.e., the therapeutic relationship) and improvement.

This chapter centers on a central hope and expectancy variable, outcome expectation (OE). In brief, OE is the prognostic belief about the effectiveness of a given course of treatment (Constantino, Vîslă, et al., 2019). It is most closely connected to Domain 2, Hope & Expectancy, in the Taxonomy of Deliberate Practice Activities in Psychotherapy (TDPA; Chow & Miller, 2022; see Appendix A, this volume). Empirically, OE has easily received the most attention among therapy-related beliefs. Because its direct influence on treatment outcomes is well established, it makes sense for therapists to understand and cultivate their OE abilities.

Of course, other types of client expectations exist, such as the roles they and their therapist will adopt and the length of treatment. Such beliefs are, however, less directly connected to clients' hopes about therapy helping them in the future. Role or duration expectancies are leveraged clinically by shaping them through role induction and attunement in the therapeutic relationship. Discussion of client pretreatment role induction and preparation, which closely corresponds to Item A in Domain 2 of the TDPA, is found in Chapter 3 ("Client Factors") of this volume. Dyadic processes related to attunement are covered in Chapter 5 ("Relationship Factors") and represented in Sections A (effective focus) and B (impact factor) of Domain 3 of the TDPA.

Whether viewed as a primary change ingredient or a necessary precursor for other change processes to work more effectively, OE is embedded in many theories of psychotherapeutic change (Constantino & Westra, 2012; Frank, 1961; Greenberg et al., 2006; Kirsch, 1990). When considered in combination with the supportive research to be reviewed next, hope and expectancy have rightful prominence in the TDPA as a focus for deliberate practice (DP).

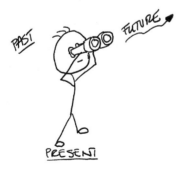

FIELD GUIDE TIP

According to Constantino, Coyne, et al. (2021), *higher* OE signifies

> a state of existing or budding optimism that psychotherapy, with its provider and surrounding context, has a personally meaningful change goal and a viable pathway to achieving it (Snyder, 2002). Conceptually, then, such a remoralized and change motivated state should facilitate psychological improvement through one's course of treatment. (p. 712)

This chapter (a) reviews the major research that supports the clinical relevance of OE in psychotherapy, (b) identifies evidence-based OE principles for clinical intervention, (c) offers suggestions for DP exercises to leverage empirically supported OE principles, and (d) highlights further practice and training-related OE resources. It is important to note the studies included in this review are drawn from the literature on adult clients, though many of the principles can be readily adapted to work with children and adolescents.

REVIEW OF RESEARCH

A client's OE can be assessed before therapy (a complete forecasting without experience of the therapist or therapy), early in treatment (a prediction with some experience of the therapist or therapy), or across treatment (a momentary prediction in the context of an evolving therapeutic relationship and treatment plan). As a dimensional variable, OE can range from extremely hopeless (e.g., "This therapy won't help me") to being very hopeful ("This treatment is going to eliminate my concerns"). There can also be grades in between, which are often represented on measures as an amount of expected improvement, such as on a scale from 0% to 100% (see Credibility/Expectancy Questionnaire [CEQ]; Devilly & Borkovec, 2000).

From treatment's outset, OE is a factor therapists should be mindful of and attempt to cultivate (if there is room for growth in the degree to which a client expects to improve from therapy) and harness (if a client's OE is already quite high). In addition, because client OE is prone to "wax and wane," it should be leveraged when high (e.g., persisting with an originally agreed-on treatment plan or approach) and responded to when low (e.g., responsively departing from the agreed-on plan; see Constantino, Coyne, & Muir, 2020; Constantino, Goodwin, et al., 2021; Coyne et al., 2019). With these objectives in mind, eight empirical findings related to cultivating and responding effectively to client OE are reviewed.

OE–Outcome Association

The finding that has put OE on the evidence-based map, so to speak, is the robust significant correlation between clients' higher pre- or early-treatment OE and outcome—specifically, greater reductions in symptomatic and/or functional impairment. A meta-analysis revealed a small but significant positive effect, with OE explaining approximately 3% of the variance in clients' posttreatment outcomes (Constantino, Vîslă, et al., 2019). To understand this figure, compare it with the contribution made by a high-quality therapeutic alliance, which explained, in a meta-analysis, about 7.5% of outcome variance (Flückiger et al., 2019). As the alliance is considered one of the most important outcome predictors, these data highlight how even seemingly moderate contributors, such as OE, can be clinically meaningful. Notably, its association with outcome in the Constantino, Vîslă, et al. (2019) meta-analysis held across different types of therapies and presenting problems, making it a principle of change clinicians should attend to and cultivate regardless of their therapeutic orientation and focus of their clinical work (see also Castonguay et al., 2019).

Moderators of the OE–Outcome Association

Three factors in the Constantino, Vîslă, et al. (2019) meta-analysis were shown to affect the strength of the link between OE and posttreatment outcome (i.e., moderation). First, client OE had an even stronger positive association with posttreatment improvement for younger versus older clients. Second, the association was stronger when OE was measured with a well-established scale versus one developed specifically for a given study. Third, and finally, client OE was a stronger predictor of outcome when therapists were using a treatment manual. The "take home" message is OE can be especially important under certain clinical circumstances.

Alliance Quality as a Mediator of the OE–Outcome Association

As with any variable–outcome correlation, it is important to understand how such an effect is transmitted (i.e., mediation). To date, one variable has robustly emerged as a mediator of the OE–outcome association: the quality of the client–therapist alliance. In a recent meta-analysis by Constantino, Coyne, et al. (2021), more hopeful OE early in care (Session 1, 2, or 3) predicted better client-rated alliance during treatment, which, in turn, predicted better posttreatment outcomes (see Figure 6.1 for a visual depiction of this mediational pathway). The indirect effect of OE on outcome through alliance quality accounted for approximately 35% of the total effect of OE on outcome. This result spotlights how relational engagement can act as a vehicle for converting a client's early optimism about treatment into therapeutic benefit. Indeed, Constantino, Coyne, et al. (2021) connected the relationship to the three central features of Snyder's (2002) hope theory:

> A quality alliance . . . embodies patient-therapist collaborative agreement on treatment targets (goals) and the tasks necessary to accomplish them (pathways), as well as an energizing emotional connection (agency; Snyder, 2002). And more than just seeing these goals and pathways as present and available, and experiencing a sense of agency in one's change process, goal theory would imply that the treatment-specific positive OE and hope would also be parlayed into devoting more psychological and behavioral resources into achieving the targets they now believe to be within their reach, to at least some degree—a type of "doing the work" of psychotherapy. (p. 712)

In light of the OE–alliance–outcome pathway to change, clinicians can have a better sense of how client OE can facilitate or hinder a shared relational process in therapy (alliance) that is known to relate to client improvement. This pathway can also manifest dyadically, with one participant's experience

FIGURE 6.1. Direct OE-Outcome Association and Indirect OE-Outcome Association Through Alliance Quality

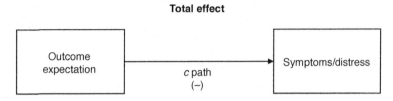

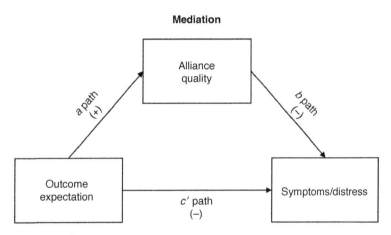

Note. The top portion of the figure shows a two-variable correlational analysis that represents the total effect of pre- or early-treatment OE on posttreatment symptoms/distress (with no mediator in the model). The results of such an analysis were reviewed in the previous section, OE-Outcome Association. The bottom portion of the figure shows each path of a mediator analysis testing alliance quality as a mediator of the OE-symptoms/distress correlation. As noted, the Constantino, Coyne, et al. (2021) meta-analysis indicated that more hopeful OE was associated with significantly lower posttreatment symptoms/distress (this total effect is labeled with a minus sign on the c′ path). Moreover, the beneficial influence of OE on posttreatment symptoms/distress was partially transmitted through better alliance quality (mediation). That is, more hopeful pre- or early-treatment OE was associated with significantly better during-treatment alliance quality (this path is labeled with a plus sign on the *a* path). In turn, better alliance quality was associated with significantly lower posttreatment symptoms/distress (this total effect is labeled with a minus sign on the *b* path).

affecting the subsequent experience of the other in the therapeutic relationship. For example, in a study of cognitive behavior therapy (CBT) for generalized anxiety disorder, greater client-rated OE after one session (measured repeatedly from Sessions 1–13) was associated with increases in therapist-rated alliance quality after the next session (measured repeatedly from Sessions 2–14), which in turn predicted lower client-rated worry in the subsequent session (measured repeatedly from Session 3 to Session 15, which was the last session; Constantino, Aviram, et al., 2020). This result suggested a client's hopeful OE can have an infectious quality on their therapist's subsequent experience of the alliance. In turn, the clinician's positive experience of the alliance can have a beneficial influence on the client's subsequent experience of worry. Bottom line? Understanding the OE-alliance-outcome path might compel therapists to routinely measure and monitor alliance and OE over time, which can provide multiple prompts for appropriate responsiveness by capitalizing on these factors when higher and explicitly addressing them when lower.

Client Characteristics That Correlate With Presenting OE

Knowing that OE is an important variable for treatment outcome has led to the study of client demographic, contextual, and clinical factors that correlate with their presenting OE. For demographic factors, female-identifying clients indicated more hopeful presenting OE than male-identifying clients in a college counseling center (Hardin & Yanico, 1983). Also, in a group therapy context, older versus younger clients presented with higher OE (Tsai et al., 2014). With regard to contextual variables, some evidence indicates clients with prior therapy experience reported more positive OE for their current group therapy than clients with no such treatment history (MacNair-Semands, 2002). As might be expected, one study suggested *satisfaction* with prior treatment is key—more satisfaction related to more hopeful OE for their current treatment for substance misuse (Tran & Bhar, 2014). In terms of clinical variables, when clients were generally more hopeful, they also reported more positive therapy-specific OE (Goldfarb, 2002; Swift et al., 2012). In addition, possessing more psychological mindedness (defined as the ability to be introspective in the service of understanding self and others) was shown to be a positive predictor of more hopeful OE (Beitel et al., 2009; Constantino et al., 2017). Finally, a meta-analysis showed that when symptoms or impairment were more severe at the start of therapy, OE was lower (Constantino et al., 2022).

Perceived Treatment Credibility-Outcome Association: Main Effect of an OE-Related Construct

A construct related to OE worth noting is client-perceived treatment credibility. It is defined as how coherent, suitable, plausible, and effective an intervention (for which at least some information has been provided) seems to a given client (Devilly & Borkovec, 2000). Although distinct from OE (because it is possible that a client could see a treatment as generally credible and yet still believe they will not benefit from it), treatment credibility is certainly in the same belief "soup," so to speak. Empirically, a small but significant positive association between credibility and improvement was identified in a recent meta-analysis (Constantino, Coyne, et al., 2019), explaining approximately 1.5% of the variance in clients' posttreatment outcomes. Notably, this association held across different client demographic variables, presenting problems, and treatment approaches. Like OE, therefore, client-perceived treatment credibility is another belief-oriented principle of change clinicians should attend to and cultivate for clinical benefit (see also Castonguay et al., 2019).

Therapist Utterances or Actions That Influence Client OE

Therapist words, utterances, and in-session actions have received a great deal of attention over the years. It is assumed, almost like magical talismans, choice, order, and timing can either harm or heal (Miller & Hubble, 2017). To date, a few lab-based studies have manipulated therapist utterances and actions to determine their impact on client OE. For example, Kazdin and Krouse (1983) found participants reported more hopeful OE after hearing an audio recorded treatment rationale that included (a) a description of the approach as "prestigious"; (b) a description of the approach as focused on affect, cognition, and behavior; (c) some theoretical jargon; and (d) examples of past successes. In another lab-based study (Horvath, 1990), participants reported more positive post-rationale OE when the recording was moderately long (vs. brief or somewhat longer). Thus, messages of moderate length could be a *sweet spot* that maximizes client comprehension through conciseness while not sacrificing the necessary details to be credible and persuasive.

Finally, a more recent clinical analog experiment (Ametrano et al., 2017) with socially anxious undergraduates compared a standard video-delivered rationale of CBT for social anxiety (control group) with one enhanced with expectancy persuasion techniques (experimental group), including those found in the aforementioned Kazdin and Krouse (1983) and Horvath (1990) studies (e.g., use of jargon and successful case vignettes). Across both conditions, the participants' OE became significantly more positive from pre- to postrationale delivery. However, no benefit was associated with the use of specific expectancy persuasion strategies. The authors argued that this lack of additive effect may have been due to the standalone potency of a clear and compelling CBT rationale for treating social anxiety. That is, in some cases, a standard rationale may be sufficient to enhance OE.

Therapist-Rated OE–Outcome Association

Although OE has been historically conceptualized and studied as a client factor, it is clear therapists also have expectations regarding the degree of success a given client will have in treatment. While research on therapist OE and client improvement is sparse, a handful of studies have provided evidence of impact over and above client OE ratings (e.g., Connor & Callahan, 2015; Swift et al., 2018). Moreover, one study added nuance to understanding the association between therapist OE and client outcome (Constantino, Aviram, et al., 2020). First, as therapist OE became more hopeful over time, clients evidenced better next-session outcomes. This demonstrates a dynamic effect of *change* in therapist OE on client improvement. Second, when therapist OE for a specific client was higher than their average OE for all clients in their caseload, those particular clients achieved better results than the therapist's average client.

Therapist Differences on Client OE

A few studies have examined whether individual therapists themselves meaningfully affect the variance in client OE. Of these studies, three have found, across different types of treatments for varied mental health concerns, some therapists foster significantly more hopeful client OE across all clients in their caseloads (Constantino, Aviram, et al., 2020; Coyne et al., 2021; Vîslă et al., 2019). One study found therapists also differed in their ability to cultivate *increases* in more hopeful client OE over the course of

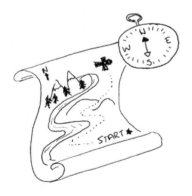

FIELD GUIDE TIP

Chapter 8 of *Better Results* (*BR*) describes and illustrates how to mine your performance data for deliberate practice opportunities.

You can put the findings on OE to use in your deliberate practice efforts by tracking your response to a question that has been shown to predict treatment outcome (scoring information can be found in Constantino, Aviram, et al., 2020).

"By the end of therapy, how much improvement in your client's (problem) do you really feel will occur?"

Begin with new clients, in time computing an average and then looking closely at the relationship between your OE and client progress and outcomes.

treatment (Vîslă et al., 2021). In sum, a small but growing research base suggests therapists can meaningfully contribute to this factor, both at any given moment and over time during treatment.

EVIDENCE-BASED PRINCIPLES RELATED TO HOPE AND EXPECTANCY FACTORS

As the research reviewed is mostly correlational, it is difficult to prescribe *definitive* ways in which therapists can clinically address clients' OE. That said, the weight of the data is such that several evidence-based principles (based on the best available science) can be identified for helping therapists cultivate and respond to their client's OE (see Table 6.1 for a concise summary of the previously reviewed research threads organized by the eight principles). Note that the principles described are drawn mainly from prior syntheses of clinical OE strategies (i.e., Ametrano et al., 2017; Constantino et al., 2012; Constantino, Coyne, et al., 2019; Constantino, Vîslă, et al., 2019; Coyne et al., 2019) and from an unpublished "expectancy persuasion" treatment manual (Constantino et al., 2006).

Principle 1: Mind Clients' Pre- and Early-Treatment OE

Therapists should regularly assess any new clients' presenting OE level to establish a baseline for how much this belief is a risk (when lower or less hopeful) or facilitative factor (when higher or more hopeful). Such measurement can be accomplished with a brief, psychometrically established self-report instrument, such as the aforementioned CEQ (Devilly & Borkovec, 2000) or the Milwaukee Psychotherapy Expectations Questionnaire (MPEQ; Norberg et al., 2011).

Second, and especially when OE is low, therapists should prioritize promoting a client's treatment-related hopefulness at the outset of therapy. Clinicians can cultivate client OE by providing a clear treatment rationale well-suited to the client's personal understanding of their presenting concerns, therapy goals, and ideas about how people change. Once the rationale is accepted, therapists can then propose and begin accompanying therapeutic strategies that are logically aligned with the rationale. To help therapists know how well this is going, they can administer the CEQ or MPEQ after presenting a treatment rationale and repeatedly through treatment. If therapists are unable to use such a measure, they should, at a minimum, assess client OE verbally.

Third, once treatment is underway and it is revealed a client's current OE is less hopeful, the clinician should consider using responsive and explicit OE-fostering strategies. For instance, they can try to deliver personalized, hope-inspiring statements, such as how the client appears to be a good candidate for the treatment before them and/or how the therapist has witnessed the treatment help clients with similar demographic and clinical characteristics in the past. Therapists can also reference in accessible language the research that supports the efficacy of psychotherapy in general and/or the selected treatment in particular.

TABLE 6.1. Summary of Findings on Outcome Expectations and Treatment Outcomes

OE finding	Level of support	Principle no.
Higher pre- or early-treatment client OE predicts better posttreatment client outcomes	MA	1
OE—outcome association stronger for younger clients	MA	2
OE—outcome association stronger when OE assessed using well-established measure	MA	2
OE—outcome association stronger when therapists use a treatment manual	MA	2
Higher pre- or early-treatment client OE predicts better therapeutic alliance quality, which predicts better post-treatment client outcomes	MA	3
Higher session one client OE predicts better therapist-rated therapeutic alliance quality the next session, which predicts better client outcome the following session	SS	3
Clients with higher symptom severity report less hopeful OE	MA	4
Clients who are more hopeful in general have higher OE	MS	4
Psychologically minded clients report more hopeful OE	MS	4
Female-identifying clients have higher OE than male-identifying clients	SS	4
Older adult clients report higher OE for group therapy than younger adult clients	SS	4
Clients with prior therapy experience report higher OE for group therapy than clients without prior treatment experience	SS	4
Clients who are more satisfied with prior treatment experiences report higher OE for treatment of substance misuse	SS	4
Higher pre- or early-treatment credibility predicts better posttreatment client outcomes	MA	5
Describing therapeutic approach as prestigious as part of the treatment rationale promotes higher client OE	SS	6
Describing therapeutic approach as broadly focused on affect, cognition, and behavior promotes higher client OE	SS	6
Using some theoretical jargon as part of the treatment rationale promotes higher client OE	SS	6
Providing examples of past successes as part of the treatment rationale promotes higher client OE	SS	6
Providing a treatment rationale of a moderate length promotes higher client OE	SS	6
Presenting a clear and compelling cognitive behavior therapy rationale for treating social anxiety promotes more hopeful client OE	SS	6
More hopeful therapist OE predicts better client outcomes	MS	7
More hopeful therapist OE at one session predicts better client outcome at the next session	SS	7
Therapists' more accurate estimation of their clients' OE predicts better posttreatment client outcome	SS	7
Some therapists foster higher client OE across all clients in their caseloads than others	MS	8
Some therapists are better able to cultivate increases over time in hopeful client OE across all clients in their caseloads than others	SS	8

Note. MA = meta-analysis; MS = multiple studies; OE = outcome expectation; SS = single study.

Conversely, therapists should consider evidence of high client OE at a given time during therapy as a "green light" to stay the current treatment course that has thus far proven to be compelling and hope inspiring. If greater hopefulness is accompanied by early client improvement (e.g., as demonstrated with a routine outcome measure), therapists will want to explicitly spotlight such progress to their clients. In doing so, therapists can frame this change as tangible evidence that the client is likely to experience additional future change as well.

Therapists should also assess and stay attentive to the possible waxing and waning of client OE throughout treatment. Again, this would ideally involve the repeated use of a brief OE measure throughout treatment. However, if unable to use such a measure, repeated verbal check-ins could be a proxy (e.g., "At this moment, how hopeful are you that this treatment approach will help you improve?"). Then, as therapists obtain such information, they should be prepared to maintain (when OE remains marked by more hopefulness) or adapt (when OE becomes less hopeful) the treatment plan accordingly.

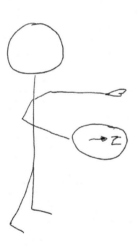

FIELD GUIDE TIP

Early on in *BR,* you were asked to create a schematic or blueprint for how you do therapy sufficiently detailed so another practitioner could understand and replicate it—literally, "step into your shoes" and work how you work (Miller et al., 2020, p. 29).

Retrieve your map, noting if, when, and how you explicitly address OE in your clinical work (e.g., from providing a clear and compelling rationale at the outset of treatment to addressing the ebb and flow of client OE throughout).

Principle 2: Mind the Circumstances Under Which OE Is Most Potent

When working with younger clients, when measuring OE with a well-established measure, and when delivering a manualized treatment, clinicians should be particularly attentive to clients' pre- and early-treatment OE level. Once aware that one or more of these contexts applies (where the connection between OE and client outcome is more potent), clinicians can draw on the same strategies outlined for Principle 1: Either try to cultivate OE when it trends toward pessimism or harness it when it trends toward hopefulness. It may be especially important under these three conditions for therapists to closely track client OE over time to capitalize on it when it waxes (e.g., persisting with a manualized therapy that continues to promote client hopefulness) and appropriately respond when it wanes (e.g., empathizing with, and perhaps shifting treatment course for, a younger client who has lost hope that the therapeutic approach will help).

Principle 3: Appreciate That OE's Effect on Outcome Is Partly Transmitted Through the Alliance

Because the therapeutic alliance helps transmit the beneficial influence of more hopeful client OE on treatment outcomes, clinicians should regularly and routinely assess both client OE and alliance quality during a course of treatment. Alliance measurement provides a proxy marker for OE level. If alliance quality has waned, for example, it would be useful to explore with the client whether this may have, at least partly, resulted from diminished hope in the effectiveness of the provider or treatment. One version of alliance repair could be to engage in OE cultivation or restoration strategies (see Principle 1). Alternatively, or in addition to these OE strategies, the clinician could engage in explicit alliance rupture-repair strategies reviewed in Chapter 5 (relationship factors); a repaired alliance could then promote better subsequent treatment outcomes.

Principle 4: Consider Known Correlates of Client OE

Therapists should familiarize themselves with client characteristics associated with OE. Beyond assessing initial risk associated with low hope or facilitating high hope, doing so can help with developing a personalized treatment plan. For clients who possess one or more risk factors for low presenting OE (e.g., male identifying, younger), a therapist might consider using first-step strategies for cultivating more initial hope (e.g., presenting a clear and compelling rationale). The strongest signal for using such interventions (without direct measurement of client OE) is when clients present with more severe impairment. Conversely, when clients present with more facilitative factors (e.g., satisfaction with prior treatment, greater psychological mindedness), it may prompt clinicians to move forward more efficiently with the treatment approach they intend to use. It is more likely that these clients already trust the therapist and are persuaded by the direction they will take (thereby capitalizing on their expectation that treatment will help them to a meaningful degree).

Principle 5: Mind Clients' Pre- or Early-Treatment Perceptions of Treatment Credibility

As with OE, at the outset of treatment with any client, therapists should attempt to foster the perceived credibility of treatment. Again, finding an individually tailored way to describe treatment that promotes a personally compelling rationale for the chosen pathway to change can go a long way toward the early establishment of credibility (e.g., Larsen & Stege, 2010a, 2010b). While providing a rationale, therapists can also

> tend to patients' verbal and nonverbal indicators that the rationale is understandable, persuasive, and interesting. Although therapists may believe that they are giving a textbook description of, say, behavioral activation for depression, a perplexed look can tell a thousand words; in this case, that behavioral activation may be unconvincing to that particular patient at that particular time. Or, at a minimum, how you are describing it may require more clarity, or a different tact. (Constantino, Coyne, et al., 2019, p. 516)

Such credibility can then be enhanced by therapists' using strategies clients perceive as consistent with their beliefs about change. Clinicians should assess credibility in addition to OE (at least verbally or with the CEQ that measures both credibility and expectancy). As with OE, such assessments should continue throughout therapy because credibility perceptions can shift.

Principle 6: Say and Do Things That Cultivate Client OE

Therapists should regularly attempt to provide a clear and strong rationale in a way that is moderate in length versus being overly wordy or underdeveloped. In addition, wording can help or hinder. Describing an approach as "prestigious," "evidence-based," and having been successful in past cases can help in fostering hope and expectation. As previously noted, clinicians should not overrely on such utterances because current evidence is not strong for their causal impact.

Principle 7: Appreciate Distinctions Between and Relations Among Therapist and Client OE

Recall, in different ways, therapists' OE can influence the degree to which a client benefits from therapy. First, as a therapist's OE dynamically increases over time, so too does the client's level of subsequent improvement. Second, higher therapist OE for a specific client relative to all their clients leads to greater-than-average improvement for that specific client (compared with that therapist's average client). As Constantino, Boswell, and Coyne (2021) noted,

> Therapists might consider both how their OE for a given patient compares to their OE for other patients in their caseload (between-patient) and how their OE for a given patient shifts over time (within-patient). Such information can help therapists respond effectively to relatively low (at, or averaged across, a specific time) or lowered (changing across time) OE. (p. 249)

Principle 8: Therapist, Know Thyself

Therapists can differ in their ability to foster their average clients' early OE or change in OE over time. Regularly measuring client OE can help therapists determine whether their clients have consistently more or less hopeful OE. If ratings tend to be middling or lower across the board, therapists should consider receiving specific training on and supervision regarding OE persuasion and expectancy interventions. And consistent with this volume's main thesis, they should deliberately practice what they learn.

EXERCISES FOR HOPE AND EXPECTANCY FACTOR SKILL DEVELOPMENT

In this section, a number of DP exercises are described, each designed to help therapists improve their OE-related skills—both those applicable at the outset or in response to variations in client OE across treatment. As in other chapters, it is assumed that you (a) are routinely monitoring your therapeutic outcomes, (b) are in possession of data sufficient to establish a reliable, evidence-based profile of your therapeutic effectiveness, (c) have completed the TDPA, (d) identified specific skill deficits in your performance related to hope and expectancy, (e) narrowed your focus to a single element within this domain on the TDPA, and (f) defined performance improvement in SMART terms (specific, measurable, achievable, relevant, and time bound) per the final instructions. Review the following exercises for those that best align with your improvement goal.

Exercise 1: Assessing OE Therapeutically

Principle: 1
Applicability: TDPA Items 2A, B, and G (also applicable to Items 1E, F, H, 3Aiii, iv, Bi, 3D, 4A, E)
Purpose
This exercise aims to increase skills in applying OE assessment in a therapeutic manner.

Task
Part 1. Begin using a brief, formal measure of OE (e.g., the OE scale of the CEQ or the MPEQ; Devilly & Borkovec, 2000; Norberg et al., 2011). Together with a colleague, coach, or supervisor, practice using the measure therapeutically. In role-plays, help the client

- give responses enabling you to gain an accurate understanding of their OE, and

- clarify the individual features of their OE—why they feel the way they do (e.g., previous experiences, your presentation, what they have heard about the treatment you are offering).

Ask the person practicing with you to enact different levels and types of OE alongside varying amounts of openness and honesty. Doing so will provide critical opportunities for enhancing your OE assessment skills as well as identifying individualized OE features to address or build on. As you did with measures of outcome and alliance, practice orienting clients to the nature and purpose of the questionnaire (e.g., creating a culture of feedback). For instance, "I am going to ask you to complete a survey that measures how hopeful you are that therapy will be helpful to you. It will let me know whether we are on the right track and help us discuss our work together. I invite you to be as open and honest as possible, even though you might feel pulled to answer in a way that would please me. Does this sound like something we could try?"

Part 2. Brainstorm questions befitting your style and therapeutic orientation for assessing and exploring client OE through conversation and test them out with a practice partner. For example, you may practice asking a direct, specific question: "I know we have discussed your therapy expectations in general, but more specifically, on a scale of 0 to 10, how much do you think the treatment I've proposed will help you with your concerns—with 0 being *not helpful at all* and 10 being *substantially helpful*?" Your partner should respond to your entreaties, providing you with an opportunity to "think on your feet." Seek feedback, reflect, and revise, and then complete the exercise again with relevant modifications to your approach.

Exercise 2: Let's Talk About Hope

Principle: 1
Applicability: TDPA Item 2A and G (also applicable to Items 1D–F, 3Aiii, iv, 3Diii, 4A, B)
Purpose
This exercise aims to build skills in opening and guiding a dialogue about client OE in the context of varying levels of hopefulness, as well as learning to do so in different, responsive ways while avoiding being overly scripted.

Task
Practice opening a discussion about the results of the expectancy measure or verbal assessment based on various possible client responses. Specifically, practice starting an OE discussion with

- a client who reports low hopefulness where remedial action may be required or
- a client reporting high hopefulness that can be leveraged for optimal benefit.

For example, you could begin practice activities by testing opening statements and questions, such as, "I noticed your score on this measure was high—does this fit with how you're feeling about how this treatment is going?" or "What seems to be helpful about this treatment right now?" You can also take time to imagine how you would respond to a client who is less hopeful by saying, "I noticed you answered this question in such a way that indicates you might be feeling that our work together may not prove helpful for you in the long run. Would you be open to discussing this further with me? I'd like to move away from those things you don't find useful."

Next, imagine various versions of what you would say to a client who answers positively, negatively, or ambiguously. Try them out with a colleague who role-plays the client. As the conversation evolves, aim to identify ways in which the treatment or its rationale could be adjusted to address low hopefulness. Conversely, use the conversation to practice identifying ways to capitalize on high hopefulness for client benefit. For maximum benefit, record and review your role-playing, limiting the exchange to 5 minutes and using your practice partner's feedback to guide successive repetitions of the exercise. Slowly increase the difficulty over time, asking your partner to use client presentations they find challenging.

Exercise 3: Just Be Curious

Principle: 1
Applicability: TDPA Items 2D–F (also applicable to Items 1G, 3Aiii, Div)
Purpose
This exercise aims to develop skills in leveraging OE when client outcomes improve. Through practice, you will learn ways of capitalizing on therapeutic successes to optimize hope and expectancy.

Task
Part 1. At the end of each day, take 5 minutes to reflect on the clients you met, paying particular attention to how you responded to reports of progress. Write down the client's name, presenting problem, what you said or did (using no more than a Twitter-length sentence), and how much time was spent on discussing progress relative to other matters discussed in the session. Continue this activity several times a week, spending no more than 20 minutes at a time. After a month, retrieve your notes and begin sorting the collection into themes (e.g., age, gender identification, level of emotional distress, diagnosis). Refine the list if needed by continuing the exercise for a few additional days.

Part 2. Recalling that DP is designed to address performance deficits, pick the theme on which you spent the *least* amount of time discussing progress, first exploring the reason for the difference and then writing out how you will be more curious in the future under such circumstances. Specifically, script how in your own words and style, you could

- elicit a clear description of the improvement from the client's perspective,
- elicit the client's reasons for the improvement,
- identify ways that treatment may have helped with this improvement (with room to discuss ways it may not have helped), and
- discuss how hopeful they feel about therapy now and possible future improvements.

Part 3. Finally, try out what you develop with a practice partner who presents either as a client who attributes improvement to the helpfulness of therapy or one who does not. Along the way, go slow, stopping to reflect whenever you encounter a challenging moment or are at a loss for words. Develop at least two alternative responses, eventually enacting these in the role play. Whatever you try out, get feedback from your practice partner on their experience as the client.

Exercise 4: Responding to Pessimism

Principle: 2
Applicability: TDPA Items 2B–D (also applicable to Items 1F, 3Aiii, 5Aii, iv)
Purpose
This exercise aims to use your clinical experiences to develop skillful responses to situations where hope and expectancy are low.

Task
Part 1. For several weeks, keep track of clients who express pessimism in the initial visits about therapy resolving their difficulties. After identifying at least two or three, pick one and devote 20 minutes to recalling your response, writing out as much of the dialogue as possible. Set what you've written aside, returning to it in your next scheduled DP period. Check your recollection, making any needed edits. Now, rewrite your comments, working to strike a balance between inspiring hope while not being overly optimistic or risking the client feeling you do not understand their situation. For example, you might begin with something like, "You've been struggling for a long time on your own, but you've come to the right place. I've been using this treatment approach for a number of years to help clients with similar concerns, and because you're motivated to explore your thought processes more in depth, it seems like a great fit for you." Next, imagine the client's response, both positive and accepting and negative and skeptical. Write responses for both possibilities. Once completed, move on to the next client. Remember, DP is a marathon, not a sprint. The point of the process is *not* "crossing the finish line" but rather reflecting on the moment-to-moment actions making up the race.

Part 2. Having rewritten your conversations with clients, role-play live with a practice partner. Begin by asking them to recall one of their own clients who presented with low OE. Have them "turn up" or "turn down" specific client attributes in, for example, a client who is moderately responsive, slightly responsive, or even unresponsive to your approach. Use your partner's feedback to refine successive trials of the hopeful initial dialogue.

Exercise 5: Developing and Refining an Effective Treatment Rationale

Principle: 2, 5, 6
Applicability: TDPA Items 2A–C, E–G (also applicable to Items 1A, F, K, 3Diii, 4A)
Purpose
In this exercise, you will design and develop a treatment rationale that fits with existing evidence and can be personalized to different client presentations.

Task

Part 1. Retrieve the schematic or blueprint you created after reading *Better Results* (*BR*; Miller et al., 2020) and refined after completing the exercises in Chapter 1 of the *Field Guide*. Locate when and how you describe your treatment rationale. If absent, write one out in clear, easily understandable language. Your rationale should include

- a statement regarding the *general* efficacy of psychotherapy (e.g., "People who go to therapy for mental health concerns are better off than 80% of those who do not");

- the research support for and a brief description of your *specific* treatment, including a basic overview of how it works and the nature of the strategies employed;

- metaphors that help to communicate the effectiveness of treatment (e.g., "Psychotherapy is as effective as coronary artery bypass surgery and has fewer side effects"); and

- your experience with the method employed and past work with people who have similar presenting concerns, histories, and/or identities.

Add or update your blueprint accordingly.

Part 2. Ask a trusted colleague to pick two or three different clients with whom they have worked, and role-play the part of a first meeting during which you deliver your rationale. Request they include clients on a spectrum from skeptical and unenthusiastic to enthusiastic and fully convinced about the benefits of therapy. Because such exchanges are information dense, spend no more than 5 to 7 minutes on the exercise. Record your practice session for later review and refinement, including any immediate feedback they provide.

Part 3. Perceptions of treatment credibility suffer when clients experience a lack of fit with the treatment rationale and plan. This portion of the exercise is focused on reengaging "at-risk" clients. Begin by reviewing your caseload, identifying any clients at risk for a negative or null outcome (e.g., less than reliable change or in the red zone on various outcome management software programs; see pages 67–69 in *BR*). Write a brief description of each, focusing specifically on who they are as individuals rather than how they are similar to other clients. Chow's (2022) "Four S" approach may be helpful in completing the process, noting (a) their sense of self (e.g., beliefs, personality, what they identify with), sparks (e.g., what they care about, what makes them come alive), significant life events (e.g., traumas, fortuitous and formulative happenings), and systems (e.g., positive and negative impactful relationships, critical environmental supports).

Next, review the treatment plan for each of these clients, noting the degree of fit with their 4 Ss. Pay particular attention to how they understand the origin and nature of their mental health concerns because this will influence what treatment approaches and activities they find credible. Modify the rationale and plan in accordance with the individual's 4 Ss and understanding of their presenting concerns. Take your time in completing the task. Devoting a few minutes each day to the exercise is likely to prove more helpful in fostering the thinking and reflecting necessary to have an impact on subsequent performance than trying to complete it in a single sitting.

Exercise 6: Addressing Correlates of Client OE

Principle: 4
Applicability: TDPA Items 2B–G (also applicable to Items 3Aiv, Ci, 4A–C)
Purpose
This exercise aims to help develop skills in identifying and addressing correlates of clients' OE.

Task
First, review your current clients, identifying those possessing features correlating with OE. Recall these include

- greater symptom or impairment severity (associated with lower OE),
- male gender identity (associated with lower OE),
- younger age (associated with higher OE),
- negative experience of previous therapy (associated with lower OE),
- greater psychological mindedness (associated with higher OE), and
- greater general hopefulness (associated with higher OE).

Next, with specific clients in mind, write how you addressed (or will address with similar clients in the future) their therapy OE. For example, with someone who has had a prior course of treatment, you might begin with a question about how satisfied they were, adding context and details to your inquiry: "Being in treatment before can be both good and bad. Research shows, for example, both can affect how a person expects to be helped. Would you be open to discussing your prior experience and if and how it might influence how helpful you expect our work together to be?"

Finally, referencing one or more of the characteristics described earlier, identify a previous client who dropped out or had a negative or null outcome, or identify a current client who is not making progress. After describing the client to your colleague, supervisor, or coach, practice delivering the responses you wrote out. Because such exchanges are information dense, spend no more than 5 to 7 minutes on the exercise. Record your practice session for later review and refinement, including any immediate feedback they provide.

Exercise 7: How Hopeful Are You?

Principle: 7
Applicability: TDPA Items 2E–G (also applicable to Items 3Biv, 4A, 5Aii, iv)
Purpose
This exercise aims to help you reflect on the way your own OE may impact your clients.

Task

At the end of the first session with every new client, rate your hope and expectation for success using the OE scale of the CEQ, the MPEQ, or a simple scaling question (e.g., 0–10; Devilly & Borkovec, 2000; Norberg et al., 2011). After a month, or when you have met each client at least three or four times, divide them into two groups—one for which you had more hopeful OE (e.g., a 7 or higher on a scale from 0 to 10) and another less hopeful (e.g., 3 or lower). Compare the alliance and outcome scores of the two groups. Should a difference be present, reflect on how your initial low OE may have influenced your therapeutic relationship and the treatment's effectiveness. Next, for each client, identify the session when your low OE began to have a negative impact. Note whether a pattern exists in terms of timing or client characteristics. Brainstorm and document alternative responses. Should no difference be found, choose to either continue gathering data for another month or reflect on the specific ways you worked with your client to (a) improve your OE or (b) integrate your positive OE into care.

FURTHER READINGS AND RESOURCES

As should be evident, OE is an evidence-based, pantheoretical, and pandiagnostic factor in psychotherapy. As such, it is worthy of attention as therapists work to hone their craft. To augment the research summary, principles, and exercises outlined in this chapter, this section provides additional readings and resources that may prove helpful as clinicians engage in their personalized DP.

Ametrano, R. M., Constantino, M. J., & Nalven, T. (2017). The influence of expectancy persuasion techniques on socially anxious analogue patients' treatment beliefs and therapeutic actions. *International Journal of Cognitive Therapy*, *10*(3), 187–205. https://doi.org/10.1521/ijct.2017.10.3.187

Constantino, M. J., Ametrano, R. M., & Greenberg, R. P. (2012). Clinician interventions and participant characteristics that foster adaptive patient expectations for psychotherapy and psychotherapeutic change. *Psychotherapy*, *49*(4), 557–569. https://doi.org/10.1037/a0029440

Constantino, M. J., Boswell, J. F., Coyne, A. E., Kraus, D. R., & Castonguay, L. G. (2017). Who works for whom and why? Integrating therapist effects analysis into psychotherapy outcome and process research. In L. G. Castonguay & C. E. Hill (Eds.), *Why are some therapists better than others? Understanding therapist effects* (pp. 55–68). American Psychological Association. https://doi.org/10.1037/0000034-004

Constantino, M. J., Coyne, A. E., Boswell, J. F., Iles, B., & Vîslă, A. (2019). Promoting treatment credibility. In J. C. Norcross & M. J. Lambert (Eds.), *Psychotherapy relationships that work: Volume 1. Evidence-based therapist contributions* (3rd ed., pp. 495–521). Oxford University Press. https://doi.org/10.1093/med-psych/9780190843953.003.0014

Constantino, M. J., Coyne, A. E., & Muir, H. J. (2020). Evidence-based therapist responsivity to disruptive clinical process. *Cognitive and Behavioral Practice*, *27*(4), 405–416. https://doi.org/10.1016/j.cbpra.2020.01.003

Constantino, M. J., Vîslă, A., Coyne, A. E., & Boswell, J. F. (2019). Cultivating positive outcome expectation. In J. C. Norcross & M. J. Lambert (Eds.), *Psychotherapy relationships that work: Volume 1. Evidence-based therapist contributions* (3rd ed., pp. 461–494). Oxford University Press. https://doi.org/10.1093/med-psych/9780190843953.003.0013

Coyne, A. E., Constantino, M. J., & Muir, H. J. (2019). Therapist responsivity to patients' early treatment beliefs and psychotherapy process. *Psychotherapy, 56*(1), 11–15. https://doi.org/10.1037/pst0000200

DeFife, J. A., & Hilsenroth, M. J. (2011). Starting off on the right foot: Common factor elements in early psychotherapy process. *Journal of Psychotherapy Integration, 21*(2), 172–191. https://doi.org/10.1037/a0023889

Muir, H. J., Coyne, A. E., Morrison, N. R., Boswell, J. F., & Constantino, M. J. (2019). Ethical implications of routine outcomes monitoring for patients, psychotherapists, and mental health care systems. *Psychotherapy, 56*(4), 459–469. https://doi.org/10.1037/pst0000246

Swift, J. K., & Derthick, A. O. (2013). Increasing hope by addressing clients' outcome expectations. *Psychotherapy, 50*(3), 284–287. https://doi.org/10.1037/a0031941

REFERENCES

Ametrano, R. M., Constantino, M. J., & Nalven, T. (2017). The influence of expectancy persuasion techniques on socially anxious analogue patients' treatment beliefs and therapeutic actions. *International Journal of Cognitive Therapy, 10*(3), 187–205. https://doi.org/10.1521/ijct.2017.10.3.187

Beitel, M., Hutz, A., Sheffield, K. M., Gunn, C., Cecero, J. J., & Barry, D. T. (2009). Do psychologically-minded clients expect more from counselling? *Psychology and Psychotherapy, 82*(4), 369–383. https://doi.org/10.1348/147608309X436711

Castonguay, L. G., Constantino, M. J., & Beutler, L. E. (Eds.). (2019). *Principles of change: How psychotherapists implement research in practice.* Oxford University Press. https://doi.org/10.1093/med-psych/9780199324729.001.0001

Chow, D. (2022, February 28). Take note of these 4 perennial factors of your clients. *Frontiers of Psychotherapist Development.* https://darylchow.com/frontiers/4s/

Chow, D., & Miller, S. D. (2022). *Taxonomy of Deliberate Practice Activities in Psychotherapy— Therapist Version* (Version 6). International Center for Clinical Excellence.

Connor, D. R., & Callahan, J. L. (2015). Impact of psychotherapist expectations on client outcomes. *Psychotherapy, 52*(3), 351–362. https://doi.org/10.1037/a0038890

Constantino, M. J., Ametrano, R. M., & Greenberg, R. P. (2012). Clinician interventions and participant characteristics that foster adaptive patient expectations for psychotherapy and psychotherapeutic change. *Psychotherapy, 49*(4), 557–569. https://doi.org/10.1037/a0029440

Constantino, M. J., Aviram, A., Coyne, A. E., Newkirk, K., Greenberg, R. P., Westra, H. A., & Antony, M. M. (2020). Dyadic, longitudinal associations among outcome expectation and alliance, and their indirect effects on patient outcome. *Journal of Counseling Psychology, 67*(1), 40–50. https://doi.org/10.1037/cou0000364

Constantino, M. J., Boswell, F. J., & Coyne, A. E. (2021). Patient, therapist, and relational factors. In M. Barkham, W. Lutz, & L. G. Castonguay (Eds.), *Bergin and Garfield's handbook of psychotherapy and behavior change* (7th ed., pp. 225–262). Wiley.

Constantino, M. J., Coyne, A. E., Boswell, J. F., Iles, B., & Vîslă, A. (2019). Promoting treatment credibility. In J. C. Norcross & M. J. Lambert (Eds.), *Psychotherapy relationships that work: Evidence-based therapist contributions* (3rd ed., Vol. 1, pp. 495–521). Oxford University Press. https://doi.org/10.1093/med-psych/9780190843953.003.0014

Constantino, M. J., Coyne, A. E., Goodwin, B. J., Vîslă, A., Flückiger, C., Muir, H. J., & Gaines, A. N. (2021). Indirect effect of patient outcome expectation on improvement through alliance quality: A meta-analysis. *Psychotherapy Research, 31*(6), 711–725. https://doi.org/10.1080/10503307.2020.1851058

Constantino, M. J., Coyne, A. E., McVicar, E. L., & Ametrano, R. M. (2017). The relative association between individual difference variables and general psychotherapy outcome expectation in socially anxious individuals. *Psychotherapy Research, 27*(5), 583–594. https://doi.org/10.1080/10503307.2016.1138336

Constantino, M. J., Coyne, A. E., & Muir, H. J. (2020). Evidence-based therapist responsivity to disruptive clinical process. *Cognitive and Behavioral Practice, 27*(4), 405–416. https://doi.org/10.1016/j.cbpra.2020.01.003

Constantino, M. J., Coyne, A. E., Muir, H. J., Gaines, A. N., Vîslă, A., & Boswell, J. F. (2022). *Patient characteristics as correlates of their psychotherapy outcome expectation: A meta-analysis and systematic review* [Manuscript in preparation]. Department of Psychological and Brain Sciences, University of Massachusetts Amherst.

Constantino, M. J., Goodwin, B. J., Muir, H. J., Coyne, A. E., & Boswell, J. F. (2021). Context-responsive psychotherapy integration applied to cognitive behavioral therapy. In J. C. Watson & H. Wiseman (Eds.), *The responsive psychotherapist: Attuning to clients in the moment* (pp. 151–169). American Psychological Association. https://doi.org/10.1037/0000240-008

Constantino, M. J., Klein, R., & Greenberg, R. P. (2006). *Guidelines for enhancing patient expectations: A companion manual to cognitive therapy for depression* [Unpublished manuscript]. Department of Psychological and Brain Sciences, University of Massachusetts at Amherst.

Constantino, M. J., Vîslă, A., Coyne, A. E., & Boswell, J. F. (2019). Cultivating positive outcome expectation. In J. C. Norcross & M. J. Lambert (Eds.), *Psychotherapy relationships that work: Evidence-based therapist contributions* (3rd ed., Vol. 1, pp. 461–494). Oxford University Press. https://doi.org/10.1093/med-psych/9780190843953.003.0013

Constantino, M. J., & Westra, H. A. (2012). An expectancy-based approach to facilitating corrective experiences in psychotherapy. In L. G. Castonguay & C. E. Hill (Eds.), *Transformation in psychotherapy: Corrective experiences across cognitive behavioral, humanistic, and psychodynamic approaches* (pp. 121–139). American Psychological Association. https://doi.org/10.1037/13747-008

Coyne, A. E., Constantino, M. J., Gaines, A. N., Laws, H. B., Westra, H. A., & Antony, M. M. (2021). Association between therapist attunement to patient outcome expectation and worry reduction in two therapies for generalized anxiety disorder. *Journal of Counseling Psychology, 68*(2), 182–193. https://doi.org/10.1037/cou0000457

Coyne, A. E., Constantino, M. J., & Muir, H. J. (2019). Therapist responsivity to patients' early treatment beliefs and psychotherapy process. *Psychotherapy, 56*(1), 11–15. https://doi.org/10.1037/pst0000200

Devilly, G. J., & Borkovec, T. D. (2000). Psychometric properties of the credibility/expectancy questionnaire. *Journal of Behavior Therapy and Experimental Psychiatry, 31*(2), 73–86. https://doi.org/10.1016/S0005-7916(00)00012-4

Flückiger, C., Del Re, A. C., Wampold, B. E., & Horvath, A. O. (2019). Alliance in adult psychotherapy. In J. C. Norcross & M. J. Lambert (Eds.), *Psychotherapy relationships that work: Evidence-based therapist contributions* (3rd ed., Vol. 1, pp. 24–78). Oxford University Press. https://doi.org/10.1093/med-psych/9780190843953.003.0002

Frank, J. D. (1961). *Persuasion and healing: A comparative study of psychotherapy*. Johns Hopkins University Press.

Goldfarb, D. E. (2002). College counseling center clients' expectations about counseling: How they relate to depression, hopelessness, and actual-ideal self-discrepancies. *Journal of College Counseling, 5*(2), 142–152. https://doi.org/10.1002/j.2161-1882.2002.tb00216.x

Greenberg, R. P., Constantino, M. J., & Bruce, N. (2006). Are patient expectations still relevant for psychotherapy process and outcome? *Clinical Psychology Review, 26*(6), 657–678. https://doi.org/10.1016/j.cpr.2005.03.002

Hardin, S. I., & Yanico, B. J. (1983). Counselor gender, type of problem, and expectations about counseling. *Journal of Counseling Psychology, 30*(2), 294–297. https://doi.org/10.1037/0022-0167.30.2.294

Horvath, P. (1990). Treatment expectancy as a function of the amount of information presented in therapeutic rationales. *Journal of Clinical Psychology, 46*(5), 636–642. https://doi.org/10.1002/1097-4679(199009)46:5<636::AID-JCLP2270460516>3.0.CO;2-U

Kazdin, A. E., & Krouse, R. (1983). The impact of variations in treatment rationales on expectancies for therapeutic change. *Behavior Therapy, 14*(5), 657–671. https://doi.org/10.1016/S0005-7894(83)80058-6

Kirsch, I. (1990). *Changing expectations: A key to effective psychotherapy.* Brooks/Cole.

Larsen, D. J., & Stege, R. (2010a). Hope-focused practices during early psychotherapy sessions: Part 1. Implicit approaches. *Journal of Psychotherapy Integration, 20*(3), 271–292. https://doi.org/10.1037/a0020820

Larsen, D. J., & Stege, R. (2010b). Hope-focused practices during early psychotherapy sessions: Part 2. Explicit approaches. *Journal of Psychotherapy Integration, 20*(3), 293–311. https://doi.org/10.1037/a0020821

MacNair-Semands, R. (2002). Predicting attendance and expectations for group therapy. *Group Dynamics, 6*(3), 219–228. https://doi.org/10.1037/1089-2699.6.3.219

Miller, S. D., & Hubble, M. A. (2017). How psychotherapy lost its magick: The art of healing in an age of science. *Psychotherapy Networker, 41*(2), 28–37, 60–61.

Miller, S. D., Hubble, M. A., & Chow, D. (2020). *Better results: Using deliberate practice to improve therapeutic effectiveness.* American Psychological Association. https://doi.org/10.1037/0000191-000

Norberg, M. M., Wetterneck, C. T., Sass, D. A., & Kanter, J. W. (2011). Development and psychometric evaluation of the Milwaukee Psychotherapy Expectations Questionnaire. *Journal of Clinical Psychology, 67*(6), 574–590. https://doi.org/10.1002/jclp.20781

Snyder, C. R. (2002). Hope theory: Rainbows in the mind. *Psychological Inquiry, 13*(4), 249–275. https://doi.org/10.1207/S15327965PLI1304_01

Swift, J. K., Derthick, A. O., & Tompkins, K. A. (2018). The relationship between trainee therapists' and clients' initial expectations and actual treatment duration and outcomes. *Practice Innovations, 3*(2), 84–93. https://doi.org/10.1037/pri0000065

Swift, J. K., Whipple, J. L., & Sandberg, P. (2012). A prediction of initial appointment attendance and initial outcome expectations. *Psychotherapy, 49*(4), 549–556. https://doi.org/10.1037/a0029441

Tran, D., & Bhar, S. (2014). Predictors for treatment expectancies among young people who attend drug and alcohol services: A pilot study. *Clinical Psychologist, 18*(1), 33–42. https://doi.org/10.1111/cp.12009

Tsai, M., Ogrodniczuk, J. S., Sochting, I., & Mirmiran, J. (2014). Forecasting success: Patients' expectations for improvement and their relations to baseline, process and outcome variables in group cognitive-behavioural therapy for depression. *Clinical Psychology & Psychotherapy, 21*(2), 97–107. https://doi.org/10.1002/cpp.1831

Vîslă, A., Constantino, M. J., & Flückiger, C. (2021). Predictors of change in patient treatment outcome expectation during cognitive-behavioral psychotherapy for generalized anxiety disorder. *Psychotherapy, 58*(2), 219–229. https://doi.org/10.1037/pst0000371

Vîslă, A., Flückiger, C., Constantino, M. J., Krieger, T., & Grosse Holtforth, M. (2019). Patient characteristics and the therapist as predictors of depressed patients' outcome expectation over time: A multilevel analysis. *Psychotherapy Research, 29*(6), 709–722. https://doi.org/10.1080/10503307.2018.1428379

7

Structural Factors

Nicholas Oleen-Junk and Noah Yulish

You learn techniques to understand principles. When you understand the principles, you will create your own techniques.

—ALAIN GEHIN, IN *ACCESSING THE HEALING POWER OF THE VAGUS NERVE*

DECISION POINT

Begin here if you have read the book, *Better Results* and

- are routinely measuring your performance *and*
- have collected sufficient data to establish a reliable, evidence-based profile of your therapeutic effectiveness *and*
- have completed the Taxonomy of Deliberate Practice Activities in Psychotherapy *and*
- need help developing deliberate practice exercises that leverage structural factors.

In this chapter, a lesser discussed but increasingly evidenced-based thera-peutic factor is conceptualized and operationalized: the structure of treatment (Duncan et al., 2010; Hubble et al., 1999; Proctor & Rosen, 1983). The purpose is to help clinicians optimize the contribution to outcome made by structural

https://doi.org/10.1037/0000358-008
The Field Guide to Better Results: Evidence-Based Exercises to Improve Therapeutic Effectiveness,
S. D. Miller, D. Chow, S. Malins, and M. A. Hubble (Editors)

elements in their work, including maintaining focus on the constituent components and associated actions important to outcome, ensuring effective pacing in and between sessions, and understanding when the services as constructed and delivered by the clinician are (and are not) working. The material that follows is divided into four sections, each specifically designed to be applicable across theoretical orientations:

- a review of the research on therapeutic structure
- a framework for conceptualizing the contribution of structure to outcome
- a presentation of evidence-based principles
- exercises for practicing the skills that improve therapeutic structure

Before proposing a conceptualization of therapeutic structure and reviewing the evidence for its effects on client outcomes, it is important to address what many view as *the* quintessence of structure in clinical work: the models and techniques used by practitioners (e.g., cognitive behavior, time-limited dynamic therapy, solution-focused, eye movement desensitization and reprocessing, interpersonal psychotherapy). While treatment models (and related theories regarding human change) are frequently the clinical topics most enthusiastically pursued by trainees and professionals, decades of sophisticated research consistently show they bear little, if any, relationship to outcome (Wampold et al., 2017; Wampold & Imel, 2015). Simply put, it is time to abandon the notion that clinicians can choose the best approach for a particular problem based on its empirical supremacy. And while it may at first seem contradictory, when properly considered, the organization of clinical activity provided by models and techniques does make an important contribution to the effectiveness of psychotherapy.

Consider first how theoretical models and techniques introduce trainees to therapy. Whether presented in introductory textbooks, video recordings of master therapists, detailed treatment manuals, or the reflections of expert therapists who have reimagined their approaches over the years (e.g., Irvin Yalom, e.g., 2017; Francine Shapiro, e.g., 2002; Neil Jacobson, e.g., Hines, 1997), models and techniques provide a sense of focus and direction (i.e., what is relevant to discuss and explore, the goals deemed important, the route therapeutic work will take, and indicators of success and failure). Thus, in this chapter, the theories, protocols, and techniques associated with specific treatment approaches are not discussed or analyzed. Instead, emphasis is placed on identifying and elucidating the structures contributing to the effectiveness of all treatment models. In so doing, the persistent, cynical, and inaccurate interpretations of the *dodo verdict* (the well-supported finding that all empirically validated psychotherapies, regardless of their specific components, produce equivalent outcomes) are avoided (see the exchange between Hofmann & Barlow, 2014, and Laska & Wampold, 2014)—interpretations that can engender either an overly strict or laissez-faire approach to training and professional development. As we show, the seemingly paradoxical nature of treatment models (i.e., high interest or importance but little direct effect on outcomes) disappears when the wisdom accumulated in their telling is balanced with practical benefits of having a structured story to go by.

From a philosophical perspective, conceptualizing *the* underlying structure of effective treatment represents, in part, "the search for the essence of the psychotherapeutic transaction" (Mendel, 1963, p. 301). This task is far from straightforward. Unlike professionals operating in what Bacon (2018) called "fundamental reality," the psychotherapist and their client work in a constructed reality. As the data supporting the dodo verdict make clear, any number of credible explanatory models and accompanying rituals may bring about wanted change. The structure of talk therapy might be contrasted with the structure of cardiology, engineering, and firefighting insofar as the former organizes the constructed world of beliefs, whereas the latter organizes the more fundamental reality of body systems, building materials, burn rates, and drafting. As such, the psychotherapist is tasked with creating and modulating the structure of treatment from client to client, session to session, and even within individual sessions. Developing an understanding of the therapeutic structure clinicians impose on their clinical work (intentionally or subconsciously) is essential to remaining flexible and responsive to varying client, therapist, and cultural factors. To give the reader a sense of both the promise and ambiguity of the subject, available research is first reviewed.

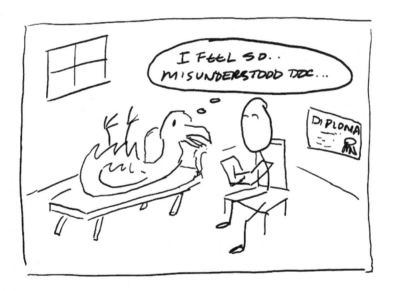

REVIEW OF RESEARCH

In research and writing, therapeutic structure is often treated as binary in nature (e.g., structured vs. unstructured), relegated to the status of a moderator variable (e.g., Baskin et al., 2003) or equated with the use of a specific psychotherapy technique or approach (e.g., structuring in client-centered therapy; Patterson, 1985). With a few notable exceptions (Duncan et al., 2010; Hubble et al., 1999), less interest and attention has been paid to structure as an independent contributor to outcome. An important early study by Grencavage and Norcross (1990) identified "treatment structures" as one of five effective ingredients shared by all therapy modalities that also included client characteristics, change processes, relationship elements, and therapist qualities. According to the authors, *treatment structures* refer to (a) techniques or rituals, (b) a focus on emotional expression and internal experiences, (c) good communication (verbal and nonverbal), (d) adherence to theory, (e) a healing setting, and (f) an explanation of therapy and participants' roles. Using more advanced statistical procedures, a later study by Tracey (2003) confirmed the importance of structure, indicating that all effective therapies (a) were theoretically consistent, (b) created positive expectations, (c) included a healer working in a healing setting, and (d) employed specific techniques. Acknowledging the sparse evidence on therapeutic structure, Tracy nonetheless argued the results reflected a need for psychotherapy to be "structured in a way that operationalizes the treatment for the client" (p. 411).

Thus, by the turn of the 21st century, an empirically informed, transtheoretical definition of therapeutic structure was beginning to take shape. By that time, psychotherapy research had already left a faint but still discernable trail of evidence indicating successful therapies had something "structural" in common. An early empirical signal that transtheoretical structural factors account for better results in therapy can be seen in a study investigating outcomes in time-limited dynamic therapy, a model that emphasizes the development of an explicit focus. Investigating the relationship between certain technical errors and outcomes, Sachs (1983) found clients' reports of a lack of focus and structure were among the errors in technique that proved the most powerful predictors of poor results. Relatedly, Weisz et al. (1995) found structural factors accounted for *better* outcomes in psychotherapy conducted with children and adolescents. Analyzing the superior outcomes achieved in research treatments relative to those conducted in clinics, the authors argued there was strong evidence that structure accounted for the difference. Briefly, their definition of structure included a preplanned set of procedures used in a particular order, sometimes guided by a manual, monitored for fidelity by direct observation or video or audio recording, and involving more specific, focused treatment methods.

In a study reviewing negative outcomes in self-administered therapy, Scogin et al. (1996) pointed to the important structural factor of preparing clients for the tasks involved in treatment as an explanation for the significantly reduced deterioration rates in the studies he analyzed. Preparation involved simply informing clients that they would be receiving a book to read as the primary therapeutic activity (p. 1088). Although the execution of most therapies involves a more nuanced implementation or facilitation of structure (more on this later), the principle remains the same: Structure helps operationalize therapy for the client (Tracey, 2003). A more detailed review of what, in the literature, is referred to as "client role preparation/induction" can be found in Chapter 3 (pp. 52–53).

A study published in 2003 by Baskin et al. provided some of the strongest, albeit indirect, evidence that the overall structure of therapy (vs. delivery of theory-specific "active" ingredients) is responsible for the outcome of treatment. Briefly, in a meta-analysis of 21 studies involving 921 clients, the researchers found bona fide psychological treatment approaches outperformed placebos largely when the latter were "structurally inequivalent" to the former ($d = 0.465$). Implicating multiple structural factors in the process, the researchers reported that when the comparison condition did *not* differ in (a) the number, length, format (i.e., group or individual), and content of sessions (i.e., whether clients were allowed to discuss topics relevant to their concerns or were restricted to general discussions); (b) the training of the therapists; and (c) the individualization of interventions to the clients, "the benefits produced by [placebo comparison groups] were largely [equivalent to] the active treatments to which they were compared (i.e., $d = 0.149$, which although statistically different from zero is negligible)" (p. 976).

The most recent evidence on the topic shows therapy is most effective when it is focused on a specified set of problems and reasonable procedures for resolving them. A meta-analysis by Yulish et al. (2017) found, for example, the extent to which a given treatment was structured to create positive expectations for clients while using specific targeted techniques (e.g., behavioral interventions for anxiety) predicted treatment efficacy ($g = .28$ for targeted symptoms; $g = -.29$ nontargeted symptoms). The results of this analysis involving 135 studies with more than 175 comparisons suggest, regardless of theoretical orientation, addressing clients' problems with focused interventions is a key structural ingredient of effective treatment.

A summary of the research on therapeutic structure is provided in Table 7.1.

The Metastructure of Effective Psychotherapy Structures

When considered together, a natural order emerges among the individual findings related to effective treatment structures. Therapeutic structures are organized along three dimensions based on their function, and help the therapist and client (a) establish the *boundaries* of the work by delimiting what is and is not helpful, (b) *sequence* its delivery to ensure predictability in manner and form, and (c) accurately *appraise* the effectiveness of the process in an ongoing and systematic fashion (see Table 7.2).

The three dimensions offer practitioners an evidence-based structure underlying the specifics of their chosen theories and methods that can aid in conceptualizing, assessing, modifying, and, as will be seen shortly, working to improve their clinical work through deliberate practice (DP). As illustrated in Figure 7.1, each dimension extends along a continuum from tight, formalized, and rigid (e.g., manualized, protocol-driven, therapist-directed services) to more informal, loosely organized, and flexible (e.g., few preplanned interventions, client directed). The *y*-axis represents the boundary dimension, indicating the

TABLE 7.1. Evidence for Transtheoretical Structural Factors That Lead to Better Outcomes

Structural factors	Evidence
Focus and structure	Clients or participants endorsed lack of focus and structure as the most important errors in technique leading to poorer outcomes (Sachs, 1983).
Techniques or rituals Focus on affect or internal experience Good communication Healing setting Explanation of therapy or roles	Content analysis of published works identifying aspects common to all therapies yielded the superordinate category of "structure" (Grencavage & Norcross, 1990).
Preparation for therapy	Clients receiving an accurate description of the intervention achieved better results in self-directed therapy than those who did not (Scogin et al., 1996).
Preplanned set of procedures Procedures used in a particular order Use of a manual Monitored for fidelity via direct observation or video or audio recording More specific focused treatment methods	Superior outcomes in youth therapy research trials versus private or public clinics is explained, in part, by structural differences (Weisz et al., 1995).
Theory consistency Positive expectations Healing setting or healer role Specific techniques	Cluster analysis of survey responses of therapy experts yielded a superordinate category, "structural factors" (Tracey, 2003).
Number and length of sessions Training of the therapist Interventions tailored to clients Topics addressed are germane Session format (e.g., group)	Meta-analysis of outcome trials revealed that holding these structural factors constant eliminates observed differences in outcome between placebo comparison groups and bona fide models of psychotherapy (Baskin et al., 2003).
Problem focus Reasonable procedures for resolving problems Creating expectations for therapy	Meta-analysis of randomized controlled trials for anxiety demonstrated these structural factors were associated with better outcomes (Yulish et al., 2017).

extent to which a given therapy remains organized around and focused on specific content and therapeutic aims. Open-ended conversations of a more diffuse nature would lie on the unstructured end, while those focusing on discrete themes with prespecified problem-resolving processes would fall on the structured side of the continuum (i.e., tightly bounded). Sequence is found on the *x*-axis, representing the extent to which elements of time, order, and format are imposed by the therapist. Following a standardized treatment protocol would, for example, be considered highly structured. By contrast, working actively to tailor services to the culture, identity, preferences, and goals of each client (see Chapters 3 and 5) would fall on the opposite end. The

TABLE 7.2. Grouping Structural Factors Along Three Dimensions of Therapeutic Structure

Dimension and function	Structural factors identified in the literature
Boundary These factors function to keep the client and therapist focused on what is helpful to delimit the bounds of the therapeutic task and provide a sense of what changes may be possible and how they could be reasonably achieved.	Focus Focus on affect or internal experience More specific and focused treatment methods Specific techniques Topics addressed are relevant Problem focus Creating expectations for therapy Positive expectations Reasonable procedures for resolving problems Theory consistency Use of a manual Training of the therapist
Sequence These factors' primary function is to establish a predictable format and culturally relevant explanation that enables clients to do things (e.g., talk, introspect, practice coping skills) that are not a part of their typical daily experience.	Techniques Preplanned set of procedures Procedures used in a particular order Number and length of sessions Session format (e.g., group) Healing setting
Appraisal These structural factors help the therapist and client to appraise the fruitfulness of their endeavor and make alterations as indicated.	Good communication Explanation of therapy and roles Preparation for therapy Interventions tailored to individual client Routine outcome monitoring Monitored for fidelity via direct observation or Video or audio recording

third and final axis, z, represents appraisal, which covers the extent to which structured procedures are implemented to, first, determine whether treatment is on track and, second, when changes are necessary to improve engagement and outcome. Using standardized measures to monitor the alliance and outcome of treatment, as described in both *Better Results* (*BR*) and this volume, would be a good example of the highly structured end of the continuum. The more traditional practice of relying on clinical judgment and occasional informal inquiries would definitely qualify as unstructured appraisal.

It is important to note that no amount of structure (i.e., high vs. low) among the three dimensions is inherently better. Rather, the "optimal" level will vary depending on the client; their presenting problem; therapist beliefs, knowledge, and skills; and the context and circumstances surrounding treatment. As a practical example, consider studies of client motivation reviewed in Chapter 3. Robust evidence shows adjusting the focus (boundary), dose (sequence), and intensity (appraisal) of treatment to the client's motivational level or "stage

FIGURE 7.1. Three-Dimensional Representation of Therapeutic Structures

Tightly
Bounded

Formal/Routine

Structured

Client-directed ◄— X ——————————————► Therapist-directed

Z

Y

Ad hoc/Implicit

Open

Unstructured

X: Sequence Dimension
Y: Boundary Dimension
Z: Appraisal Dimension

of change" is associated with more engagement and better outcomes (Krebs et al., 2018; Norcross et al., 2011). In this way, as therapy progresses, keeping the three dimensions in mind can help practitioners be more responsive to the individual client. In addition, when used in combination with one's outcome data, specific DP objectives might become apparent:

- Is there a mismatch between the client's stage of change and the dose (sequence) and intensity (appraisal) of the work with those who drop out of treatment?

- Do clients with poorer outcomes or alliance scores have more (or less) structure along one or more dimensions (boundary, sequence, and appraisal)?

- Are particular clients, presenting problems, or treatment circumstances associated with more mismatches?

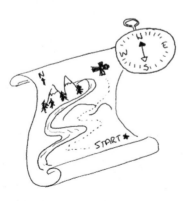

FIELD GUIDE TIP

"Certain therapists are more effective than others . . . because [they are] appropriately responsive . . . providing each client with a different, individually tailored treatment" (Stiles & Horvath, 2017, p. 71).

Ineffective Psychotherapy Structures

Some decisions therapists make regarding the structure of their work, while popular and intended to improve engagement and effectiveness, are not actually supported by the evidence. As one example, consider the popularity of manuals and diagnostic-specific treatment protocols. Here, as suggested at the outset of this chapter, the data are clear. First, degree of adherence—how closely a therapist follows directions—is not associated with outcome (Boswell et al., 2013; Wampold & Imel, 2015; Webb et al., 2010). Second, as reviewed in detail in *BR*, attempts to improve effectiveness via the creation of a psychological formulary—official lists of specific treatments for specific disorders—have failed to result in any improvement over the last 5 decades (Miller et al., 2020). In fact, clinician competence in conducting specific types of therapy for particular diagnoses has not been "found to be related to patient outcome and indeed . . . estimates of their effects [are] very close to zero" (Webb et al., 2010, p. 207). As an example, imagine a physician who interrogated every patient in the same way, always used the same set of lab tests, and prescribed medications solely on the basis of administrative policies. The intuitive grotesqueness of this hypothetical form of medicine equally applies to the practice of psychotherapy. Simply put, blindly applying interventions based on a single criterion (i.e., psychiatric diagnosis) regardless of the personal characteristics, identity, and preferences of the client does *not* work.

At the same time, the evidence shows a therapy with minimal structure can also be unhelpful (Yulish et al., 2017). One clear example of this lies in the tendency of therapists to rely too heavily on their own and clients' preferences when it comes to ending treatment. Consider a study in which practitioners were interviewed in an attempt to develop guidelines for structuring the termination process (Kramer, 1986). The results showed many practitioners, citing autonomy, relied on (e.g., trusted) their clients to bring up the issue on their own. In cases where therapist and client disagreed, therapists ignored their clients' position and encouraged them to continue. Planning for the end of therapy adds the elements of effective structure, reviewed earlier, to the termination process, promoting both a greater sense of shared focus (boundary) and time-oriented expectations (appraisal). Such structures are clearly important because research shows highly effective therapists have more planned terminations than their more average colleagues (Chow et al., 2015).

Kramer (1986) offered four guidelines for structuring termination: (a) discussing termination at the outset of therapy (e.g., negotiating a shared vision of successful completion), (b) being aware of cues that the therapeutic relationship is changing (e.g., clients require less input, clients behave more like peers, in-session frequency is reduced), (c) providing a structured review of treatment progress and process, and (d) introducing an open-door policy following the suspension of regular meetings (i.e., creating a sense that the work of therapy is ongoing). A later study by Norcross et al. (2017) confirmed and extended Kramer's early suggestions. On the basis of a factor analysis of nearly 80 termination-related tasks identified by expert practitioners, Norcross et al. identified a set of five structure-related termination guidelines: (a) orienting the client toward future growth, (b) explicitly preparing for termination, (c) consolidating gains achieved, (d) expressing pride in the client's progress, and (e) having mutuality in the relationship.

Summary and Conclusions

It might be ideal if therapists could refer to a set of proven structural elements (e.g., techniques, protocols, strategies), invariably leading to better results. However, evidence to date indicates clinical decision making is better guided by adopting the higher level of abstraction offered by the three dimensions of therapeutic structure outlined previously. Because the set of credible and effective methods is likely infinite—especially given consistent findings of equivalence between rival approaches—this conceptualization of structure facilitates flexibility while maintaining the organization and direction research shows is essential for success (Chen et al., 2020; Hipol & Deacon, 2013; Katz et al., 2019; Levitt et al., 2016; Mohr, 1995; Saidipour, 2021; van Minnen et al., 2010; Waller, 2009; Waller & Turner, 2016).

EVIDENCE-BASED PRINCIPLES RELATED TO STRUCTURAL FACTORS

With the evidence at hand, five principles for organizing and guiding DP activities related to improving therapy structure are proposed: (a) craft smarter starts to therapy; (b) avoid unhelpful structuring activities; (c) know your work; (d) know that this, too, shall end; and (e) use data wisely. Each connects specific, evidence-derived guidance to one of the three transtheoretical dimensions of therapy structure (boundary, sequence, and appraisal).

Principle 1: Craft Smarter Starts to Therapy (Sequence Dimension)

When it comes to structuring therapeutic work, the counsel offered in the song "Do Re Mi" from the classic movie *The Sound of Music* is spot on: "Let's start at the very beginning, a very good place to start." Shaping expectations about the content, aims, and conduct of the work should begin at the very first contact with the client (e.g., screening phone call, intake session). Conveying warmth (e.g., understanding, concern, hope) while establishing the boundaries of care not only sets the stage for clients returning for subsequent visits but also honors their decision to enter therapy.

Scripting a cogent and concise way of describing how you conduct therapy to novice and familiar clients is sound practice. Metaphors are one way to facilitate comprehension of such potentially complex information. Think, for example, of how you would explain flying on a commercial jet to someone who had never been on a plane. What would be essential to communicate about the experience from booking to boarding? Which aspects of the flight are more or less important (e.g., waiting in line, the safety demonstration, turbulence, drinks and snacks, bathrooms) to ensuring a pleasant and successful journey? What difficulties and challenges are most important to know about and anticipate (e.g., cancellations, rebooking, fees)? While a nearly limitless number of potential avenues for describing and discussing the experience exists, suffice it to say you cannot cover them all. Research and experience suggest a number of essential aspects:

- The topics addressed in therapy can be difficult. "To avoid client deception," Levitt et al. (2006) advised, "explicitly communicate the etiquette of therapy as one in which painful experience needs to be discussed, that therapists wish not to be protected, and the importance of talking about topics that might be threatening or invite disapproval" (p. 319).

- Work outside of sessions may be required. Because a large portion of outcome is due to extratherapeutic factors, what occurs outside the consulting room is essential to success (Duncan et al., 2010; Hubble et al., 1999; Levitt et al., 2006; Swift & Parkin, 2017; see also Chapter 3, this volume).

- Collaboration is key. David Orlinsky and colleagues (2004) argued that the client's participation in therapy is the most important factor influencing outcome and that over 40 years of psychotherapy establishes this as a fact. Accordingly, talking with clients on an ongoing basis about what they are willing to do and why it is important is critical.

- Both client and therapist have essential roles. Clients determine the destination. Therapists provide guidance and direction. "Allowing the client to set goals is experienced as empowering," Levitt et al. (2006) noted; however, "when mired in unimportant topics, clients want therapists to provide direction after checking for client's consent" (p. 319).

Principle 2: Avoid Unhelpful Structuring Activities (Boundary Dimension)

Certain ways of being (e.g., rigid, distant, critical, uncertain, overly solicitous) and particular patterns of therapist behavior (e.g., overstructuring, unyielding interpretations, inappropriate self-disclosure, talking too much or too little) are associated with alliance ruptures and poorer outcomes (Ackerman & Hilsenroth, 2001; see also Chapter 5, this volume). One reliable sign therapists may be engaging in such unhelpful structuring activities is when they attribute the resulting low levels of participation or a lack of progress *to the client*. This often appears in the form of invoking client motivational levels, citing resistance, adopting increasingly complex and severe diagnostic formulations, or what Duncan et al. (1997) referred to as *theory countertransference*—the tendency to fit clients into the therapist's preferred theory rather than closely scrutinizing their own contribution to any impasse.

Principle 3: Know Your Work (Sequence Dimension)

The expertise literature makes clear that the longer one is engaged in a particular endeavor, the less aware they become of their decision-making processes and actions (Chi, 2006; Tracey et al., 2014). Automaticity, as the process is referred to, is both good and bad. On the one hand, it is a sign that a new, higher level of control over one's performance has been attained, allowing us to devote scarce cognitive resources elsewhere. On the other hand, such proficiency typically comes at the expense of learning and improvement. As a result, improvement in performance generally begins to stall and even deteriorate. Working purposefully to counteract the loss of conscious control over behavior that occurs naturally with the mastery of specific skills is at the very heart of DP.

With time and experience, most practitioners develop an implicit sense of how therapy ought to flow as well as ideas of when it is getting off track. Unfortunately, research shows that this "gut feel" is off more of the time than we realize (Waller & Turner, 2016). Developing an explicit framework of how one works—a step-by-step map detailing how one's intuitions, beliefs, and theories connect to the sequence of events in the consulting room with clients—not only ensures consistency, predictability, and safety but is also helpful when attempting to identify where specific intentional adjustments in the flow of the work could be made to improve engagement and effect.

Principle 4: This, Too, Shall End (Sequence Dimension)

This variation on the popular saying serves as a reminder that endings in therapy are important. Unfortunately, like death, it is not the most popular subject. Some therapists, feeling the pull to maintain contact, are less structured in their approach, rarely broaching the topic and keeping the door open for unlimited visits. Others, following a predetermined treatment plan or working in certain treatment settings (e.g., close-ended groups, inpatient or residential programs), may "graduate" clients once delivery of the standardized protocol has been made or a requisite amount of time has passed.

Available evidence shows the way termination is introduced, discussed, and structured throughout therapy can have an important impact on outcome. Not infrequently, transitions are the reason people seek out a therapist. Therefore, it is important clinicians model appropriate behaviors regarding that part of the sequence of therapeutic work surrounding the end of contact. Building in a shared sense of the scarcity of time throughout the work can be the impetus for clients taking advantage of therapy.

Principle 5: Use Data Wisely (Appraisal Dimension)

It goes without saying that the first step in appraising one's performance is collecting relevant data. Readers of *BR* and this field guide know routinely monitoring the quality of their relationships and effectiveness of their work are key components of professional development and DP. In terms of structure, this not only means administering standardized assessments of outcome and alliance but also having well-defined, step-by-step processes in place for integrating them into treatment. Research shows different structures have different impacts on outcome, with those adopting a more therapeutic approach regarding the monitoring of their work obtaining greater outcome improvements (Goldberg, Babins-Wagner, et al., 2016; Goldberg, Rousmaniere, et al., 2016). No one would expect the introduction of a stopwatch to improve the ability or speed of runners or a stethoscope to improve heart functioning (Miller, 2018). Simply put, it is how the information provided by such tools is put to use that matters. Therapists do well when they create structures around what and how data are collected and used to appraise their performance, adjust therapeutic activities, and communicate with clients in a way that fosters maximum participation in treatment.

EXERCISES FOR STRUCTURAL FACTORS SKILL DEVELOPMENT

To have an impact, DP efforts must be focused on reaching for performance objectives just beyond an individual's present abilities. That means before selecting an exercise from the following list, it is essential that you have taken the time to (a) routinely measure your performance; (b) collect sufficient data to establish a reliable, evidence-based profile of your therapeutic effectiveness; (c) complete the Taxonomy of Deliberate Practice Activities in Psychotherapy (TDPA; Chow & Miller, 2022; see Appendix A, this volume); (d) determine a deficit exists related to the operation of structural factors in your work; (e) narrow your focus to a single element within this domain on the TDPA; and (f) define that performance improvement objective in SMART terms (specific, measurable, achievable, relevant, time bound). Once these steps are completed, simply review the suggested exercises, looking for the one that aligns most closely with your goal. Should none of the exercises speak directly to your specific objective, Chapter 2 provides guidance for developing your own. It describes a process for using the TDPA in combination with your data to develop a "learning project," ultimately resulting in individualized DP exercises.

Exercise 1: Using the Metastructure of Therapeutic Structure for Self-Assessment

Principle: 1–5
Applicability: TDPA Items 1 A to N
Purpose
This exercise uses the metastructure dimensions presented in the chapter to help you assess strengths and weaknesses in the way you leverage structural factors for therapeutic benefit.

Task

Table 7.3 presents questions to help clinicians identify and clarify how they impose therapeutic structure in their clinical work. Following each question are examples of client and therapist behaviors that may signal a need to improve or adjust structure to maximize fit and effect. As can be seen, beside each set of example behaviors is a list of strategies for improving therapeutic structure. Use the following steps to help you identify your learning edge and activities that may enhance your practice:

1. Using your alliance and outcome data, create a list of clients who have not benefited from therapy with you.
2. With such clients in mind, review the dimensions, questions, and behaviors listed in Table 7.3.
3. Identify any trends, behaviors, and/or strategies that come up or are missed more frequently.
4. Use your findings from this exercise to guide the focus of your DP.

Exercise 2: Using Metaphors

Principle: 1
Applicability: TDPA Items 1 A to C
Purpose
This exercise aims to help you develop clear and simple explanations about the process of therapy and its structures using metaphors.

Task

Part 1. Script a metaphor for how you do therapy, preferably one that highlights the interactive and collaborative nature of the process. An example might be renovating a house with a contractor, another a glacial expedition with a guide. What is important is that your metaphor captures how you actually work (e.g., your blueprint), as well as being consistent with your theoretical approach. Once done, test your metaphor with a coach or practice partner. As you gain confidence, rachet up the difficulty by asking your coach or practice partner to present in more challenging ways. Consider adaptations for different presentations and needs.

Part 2. Build on the metaphor developed in the previous task by developing structures for communicating the roles and processes of therapy. With your script in hand, add elements related to roles and expectations. Consider, for example, how your metaphor captures

- the role of the therapist (e.g., honest, caring, interested);
- the role of the client (e.g., work outside of the session, the value in addressing painful experiences);
- the need for client feedback regarding interventions, homework, and progress; and
- the indicators of success, failure, and completion of therapy.

Once completed, test your additions with a practice partner or coach. Use your outcome data to identify any client groups or presentations who have been

TABLE 7.3. How to Assess Therapeutic Structure

Boundary dimension	

1. How do you establish and maintain focus in a session?

Consider more structure if or when	Structural strategies for focus
• clients are uncertain about what to share in therapy	• Identify barriers to establishing a helpful focus.
• progress notes do not reflect a clear session focus	• Explain benefits of narrowing focus to topics that directly impact client functioning.
• therapist is bored or confused	
• there is lack of client-identified progress	• Provide psychoeducation regarding potential avoidance or psychological defenses.
	• Examine therapist resistance to addressing a clearer focal point in therapy.

2. How do you communicate hopes for therapy success while managing unrealistic expectations?

Consider more structure if or when	Structural strategies for therapy preparation
• client doubts change is possible	• Provide a clear and theoretically consistent explanation for how interventions lead to change.
• client has unrealistic expectations about change (e.g., eliminate all my anxiety)	
• client fears becoming overwhelmed should certain topics be broached	• Provide a theoretically consistent explanation for why certain things are not helpful in therapy.
	• Share examples of how others have responded to interventions and how to manage feelings of overwhelm.

3. How do you remain theoretically consistent and ensure interventions seem reasonable to the client?

Consider more structure if or when	Structural strategies for logical coherency
• client notes apparent contradictions in therapist's beliefs or explanations for problems	• Acknowledge contradictions and work with client (perhaps at a higher or lower level of abstraction) to reconcile apparent or problematic contradictions.
• therapist feels particularly vulnerable to client's intellectual challenges	• Help client articulate their own theories about change or behavior and make efforts to tailor conceptualizations to their narrative framework.
• client appears to be feigning effort (i.e., "going through the motions")	

Sequence dimension	

1. How do you start an initial session and subsequent sessions?

Consider more structure if or when	Structural strategies for initiating sessions
• client is confused about how to start	• Offer client examples of how an intake and subsequent sessions can unfold.
• therapist feels apprehension at the beginning of sessions with a particular client	• Collaborate with client to establish a routine at the beginning of sessions.
• client reports anxiety before sessions	• Improve consistency at the outset of sessions (note that less structure can also facilitate session starts).
• there are repeated occurrences of important disclosures at the end of session	

(continues)

TABLE 7.3. How to Assess Therapeutic Structure (*Continued*)

2. How do you close sessions?

Consider more structure if or when	Structural strategies for better closings
• there are repeated occurrences of important disclosures at the end of sessions	• Signal to the client that time is running low before time has expired and get comfortable interrupting.
• there is anxious talkativeness in the final moments of the session	• Share theory-consistent reasoning for boundaries around session time.
• there are apparent efforts to extend the session beyond the time limits (therapist or client)	• Offer suggestions about how to process thoughts and feelings that emerge at the end of the session (i.e., strategies for reflection and consolidation in between sessions).

3. How do you ensure continuity between sessions?

Consider more structure if or when	Structural strategies for continuity
• client does not complete intersession goals or tasks (e.g., "homework")	• Summarize the content of sessions and draw back to the key therapeutic focus of the work.
• therapist and client forget to follow-up on themes addressed in previous sessions	• Begin sessions with a summary of the key content from the previous session and link to key therapeutic focal targets.
• client misses sessions	• Support the client to summarize their understanding of what each session has meant for them and therapeutic aims as they see them.

Appraisal dimension

1. How do you elicit detailed and nuanced feedback in sessions?

Consider more structure if or when	Structural strategies for continuity
• it is unclear whether clients are progressing and why	• Develop and use strategies to repair ruptures in the alliance.
• routine outcome monitoring identifies that little therapeutic progress is being made	• Develop and apply structured methods for addressing nonimprovement in therapy.
• routine monitoring identifies a lower-than-expected client-rated therapeutic relationship	• Create time at the end of each session to review and appraise the session from both client and therapist perspective, specifically eliciting critical feedback.

2. How do you change your way of working in response to client feedback?

Consider more structure if or when	Structural strategies for continuity
• client feedback indicates that therapy is helpful, but they worry about when sessions finish	• Build structured ways to respond to client feedback (both positive and negative) that builds on progress and addresses problems.
• client identifies that they are unclear on the aims or goals of therapy	• Construct systems that help to collaboratively identify, refine, and agree on therapeutic goals.
• client feedback highlights that therapy is not having the desired impact on symptoms or functioning	

more likely to drop out of therapy or experience a lack of progress. Consider how you could modify your metaphor to engage better and help these specific client groups.

Part 3. Further refine your metaphor, distilling the content to its core elements for ultra-brief communication. With your metaphor in hand, pretend you are in an elevator with a new client. Using the timer on your mobile phone, deliver your pitch as written. Note the time. Without speaking faster, work to convey the key elements in 45 seconds or less. In service of clarity, practice providing your refined message to five different people, including at least one child, one colleague, and one person demographically different from yourself (e.g., in gender, culture, sexual orientation, socioeconomic status). Next, using your outcome data, first identify clients who dropped out after the first or second visit. Consider how you might have modified your message to keep them engaged, writing down different possibilities.

Exercise 3: Mapping Your Flow

Principle: 3
Applicability: TDPA Items 1 I–K
Purpose
Selecting, sequencing, and individualizing interventions are key aspects of therapeutic structure. This exercise is designed to help you refine the way these elements work in your clinical practice.

Task
Early on in *BR*, you were asked to create a schematic or blueprint for how you do therapy sufficiently detailed so another practitioner could understand and replicate it—literally, "step into your shoes" and work how you work (Miller et al., 2020, p. 29). The purpose of the activity was to make it easy to pinpoint where to intervene as opportunities for improving your effectiveness are identified by analyzing your performance data. If you have not yet completed a blueprint, turn to pages 18–20 in Chapter 1, this volume, for updated, step-by-step directions.

Next, using your outcome data, build a list of clients who did not improve while in therapy with you. With your blueprint in hand, review the work you did with each client, noting any recurring themes or mismatches among the three dimensions of therapeutic structure (e.g., boundary, sequence, and appraisal). Consider what changes or nuances need to be added to your map to more effectively structure therapy for these clients.

Exercise 4: When Therapists Drift

Principle: 2
Applicability: TDPA Items 1F, H–K
Purpose
This exercise aims to help therapists address some of the key barriers to effectively applying structure in therapy.

Task

Using your outcome or alliance data, identify one client for whom therapeutic benefit was limited. Review your case notes for each session, noting where your intended interventions or approach did not go as you hoped. Consider the following questions (derived from Waller & Turner, 2016):

- To what extent did you fully use the therapeutic intervention chosen and associated structure? Consider specifically whether you drifted from in vivo (fully experiencing) to in sensu (giving a sense of rather than supporting full experiencing).

- How did the following factors affect the way you used therapeutic techniques in the work?

  - **feedback from the client:** Was feedback sought on the client's experience of the therapeutic activity? If so, was your reaction proportionate and responsive to feedback?

  - **the client's beliefs:** To what extent did the client understand the rationale behind the activity, how it was expected to work, what they might experience in the process, and the possible outcomes?

  - **the client's emotions:** Was your response to the client's emotional experience proportionate and appropriate? Were you happy that any adjustments made were the best fit for how the client was feeling and what they could manage?

  - **the therapist's emotions:** From reviewing the session, can you gain a sense of how your own emotions may have affected the way you applied structured methods and techniques? What helped, and what hindered?

  - **the therapist's beliefs:** How did your own beliefs affect the way you approached this therapeutic activity? Are there ideas about the methods that might have prevented you from using the technique more effectively?

Once you have reviewed the sessions as described, work to identify one key learning objective. Depending on your answers to the foregoing questions, it could be about helping the client to understand the process of the activity before starting or perhaps giving structured choices for how treatment can be adapted when necessary. Recalling the advice offered in *BR* that it's "never too late to have a good session" (see pages 165–166), imagine what you would do differently if given the chance for a do-over, being as specific as possible.

Exercise 5: Finishing Strong

Principle: 4
Applicability: TDPA Items 1 A, F–I
Purpose
Depending on one's theoretical orientation, the structure of therapy endings will look different. Regardless, as reviewed in this chapter, research shows

successful completions of treatment incorporate similar elements and pacing. This exercise explores how the structural elements identified as important to effective endings operate in your therapeutic practice.

Task

Part 1. Norcross et al. (2017) identified certain structural elements central to effective endings: (a) explicitly preparing for termination, (b) orienting the client toward future growth, (c) consolidating gains achieved, (d) expressing pride in the client's progress, and (e) having mutuality in the relationship. For 1 month, keep a journal of your reflections on how you address each of these factors in your clinical practice. Consider the following questions, for example, regarding how you

- explicitly prepare for termination
  - How do you talk about termination in the first session, middle sessions, and when approaching an actual termination?
  - How do you connect goals to endings? (e.g., "How will we know therapy is complete?" or "How would you want this goal to look 12 sessions or a year from now?")
  - How do your personal needs account for how you do endings?

- orient the client toward future growth
  - How do you prepare the client for approaching future psychological concerns without you?
  - How do you convey to the client that growth and change are continuous, never-ending processes?
  - How do you speak to the client about problems or goals yet to achieve without sounding critical or dashing confidence and hope?

- consolidate gains achieved
  - How do you communicate about the progress clients have made in treatment?

- express pride in the client's progress
  - In what ways do you share your authentic feelings with clients regarding their progress?
  - Do you notice any patterns with specific clients or presenting concerns where you struggle to express such pride?

- work toward mutuality in the relationship
  - How do you support the client's independence, sense of self-confidence, and ability to solve problems in the future?
  - How do you foster a sense of equality in the relationship?

Part 2. Using your outcome data, identify five clients with whom the ending of treatment could have been improved. These might include the following:

- unplanned endings
- endings where the client reported being unprepared for termination
- episodes of therapy that seemed to continue for longer than necessary

Using paper and pencil or your favorite note-taking software, list each client by name. Next, note which of the following evidence-based approaches to structuring the ending of therapy were missing: (a) termination discussed at the outset of therapy, (b) routinely connecting therapeutic activities during treatment to the desired goal for services, (c) structured reviews of progress throughout therapy, (d) explicit mentions from the outset of treatment regarding the potential for growth beyond therapy, (e) sufficient planning for and discussion of termination before the final visit, and (f) discussion and affirmation of client improvement, including links being made to the impact of progress on posttherapy functioning.

Sort for themes, noting whether any patterns in your structure of therapeutic endings are reliably associated with a higher rate of dropout, unplanned terminations, poorer outcomes, or therapies that continue despite a lack of measurable progress. Adjust your therapy blueprint to include the missing activities at the appropriate moments during treatment.

Exercise 6: Making Data Collection Structurally Therapeutic

Principle: 5
Applicability: TDPA items 1 D–F
Purpose
This exercise aims to help therapists develop the therapeutic structure needed to sustain the use of outcome and alliance measures, even in challenging clinical situations.

Task
Next, you will find five challenging clinical scenarios related to the appraisal dimension of therapeutic structure. Taking one example per week, consider the structure you would bring to address the examples in a therapeutic manner, particularly considering how they connect to your theoretical orientation and treatment experience.

It is important not to rush the process. Let the scenarios percolate in the "back of your mind" throughout the day, keeping notes about the thoughts, feelings, and reactions that occur to you while simultaneously resisting the temptation to "solve the puzzle." The evidence indicates mulling over ideas allows us to make deeper, more nuanced connections between experiences and ideas that, in turn, increase the possibilities for creative action. When able, for each scenario, be specific about what you would focus on (boundary), when you would focus on it (sequence), and how you would continue to seek feedback through the administration and discussion of standard measures along the way (appraisal).

Scenario 1. You have been incorporating assessments into your clinical work for a year. You get a new client who tells you in the first session they are not particularly interested in doing assessments at the beginning and end of therapy because they are a waste of time. They indicate that if you insist on using the tools, they will either refuse to fill them out or answer the items randomly.

Scenario 2. A client you have been working with for several visits completes the outcome measure in a manner that suggests significant improvement since their last session. As you inquire about the change in scores, the client breaks into tears describing the last week as "the worst period in [their] life."

Scenario 3. On asking a client to complete the outcome measure you routinely use to assess progress, they cursorily mark all the items the same way (e.g., high or low).

Scenario 4. Your work with a client has been going fairly well; you have been conducting a structured, protocol-driven treatment. Regular assessments over the course of care have shown steady progress. At what is the final visit, the client expresses frustration about having to end therapy merely "because the preplanned number of sessions have been conducted." They insist that, despite their improved scores, they continue to feel miserable.

Scenario 5. Looking back over your clients over the last month, identify those with whom you have done your best to adjust to their structural requests (e.g., focus, scheduling, assessment of progress) but who continue to make little or no progress (poor outcome scores, missed sessions, low levels of engagement). Pick one and consider which structural adjustments are next, including ending treatment, referring to another provider or setting, or increasing the dose or intensity of services.

FURTHER READINGS AND RESOURCES

This chapter reviewed the available research, identified evidence-based principles, and suggested DP exercises for working with structural factors in psychotherapy. Additional research and recommendations can be found in the following:

- Particularly approachable for its concise storytelling and practical advice, Irvin Yalom's (2002) book *The Gift of Therapy: An Open Letter to a New Generation of Therapists and Their Patients* (HarperCollins) is chock-full of insights for therapists striving to improve various structural elements in their work.

Specifically, Chapters 27, 29–33, 36, 47–51, 59, 62, 65, and 73 focus on the boundary dimension; Chapters 14–23, 52, 56, 60, and 69 focus on the sequence dimension; and Chapters 11, 13, 20, 24, 37–40, 53, and 54 focus on the appraisal dimension.

- Principle 3 (know your work) invites clinicians to be more intentional about the flow of their work and how it influences client interactions. Even the most client-centered and present-focused therapists develop implicit patterns (or rituals) that govern sessions and decision making. To understand more about the importance of ritual in psychotherapy (sequence dimension, primarily), see the following:

  Moore, R. L. (1983). Contemporary psychotherapy as ritual process: An initial reconnaissance. *Zygon, 18*(3), 283–294. https://doi.org/10.1111/j.1467-9744.1983.tb00515.x.

  Al-Krenawi, A. (1999). An overview of rituals in Western therapies and intervention: Argument for their use in cross-cultural therapy. *International Journal for the Advancement of Counseling, 21*, 3–17. https://doi.org/10.1023/A:1005311925402

- For an excellent discussion of strategies and considerations related to Principle 1 (craft smarter starts to therapy), we recommend Daryl Chow's (2018) *The First Kiss: Undoing the Intake Model and Igniting the First Sessions in Psychotherapy* (Correlate Press).

- As noted in Principle 2 (avoid unhelpful structuring activities), when a therapist attributes stagnation or regression *to the client*, it can be a sign that structuring activities are not tailored to more productive therapeutic foci. For a discussion on evidence-based decision making regarding session focus (i.e., client resources vs. client problems), see

  Smith, E. C., & Grawe, K. (2005). Which therapeutic mechanisms work when? A step towards the formulation of empirically validated guidelines for therapists' session-to-session decisions. *Clinical Psychology and Psychotherapy, 12*(2), 112–123. https://doi.org/10.1002/cpp.427

REFERENCES

Ackerman, S. J., & Hilsenroth, M. J. (2001). A review of therapist characteristics and techniques negatively impacting the therapeutic alliance. *Psychotherapy, 38*(2), 171–185. https://doi.org/10.1037/0033-3204.38.2.171

Bacon, S. (2018). *Practicing psychotherapy in constructed reality: Ritual, charisma, and enhanced client outcomes.* Lexington Books/Rowman & Littlefield.

Baskin, T. W., Tierney, S. C., Minami, T., & Wampold, B. E. (2003). Establishing specificity in psychotherapy: A meta-analysis of structural equivalence of placebo controls. *Journal of Consulting and Clinical Psychology, 71*(6), 973–979. https://doi.org/10.1037/0022-006X.71.6.973

Boswell, J. F., Gallagher, M. W., Sauer-Zavala, S. E., Bullis, J., Gorman, J. M., Shear, M. K., Woods, S., & Barlow, D. H. (2013). Patient characteristics and variability in adherence and competence in cognitive-behavioral therapy for panic disorder. *Journal of Consulting and Clinical Psychology, 81*(3), 443–454. https://doi.org/10.1037/a0031437

Chen, R., Rafaeli, E., Ziv-Beiman, S., Bar-Kalifa, E., Solomonov, N., Barber, J. P., Peri, T., & Atzil-Slonim, D. (2020). Therapeutic technique diversity is linked to quality of working alliance and client functioning following alliance ruptures. *Journal of Consulting and Clinical Psychology, 88*(9), 844–858. https://doi.org/10.1037/ccp0000490

Chi, M. T. H. (2006). Two approaches to the study of experts' characteristics. In K. A. Ericsson (Ed.), *The Cambridge handbook of expertise and expert performance* (pp. 21–30). Cambridge University Press. https://doi.org/10.1017/CBO9780511816796.002

Chow, D., & Miller, S. D. (2022). *Taxonomy of Deliberate Practice Activities in Psychotherapy—Therapist Version* (Version 6). International Center for Clinical Excellence.

Chow, D. L., Miller, S. D., Seidel, J. A., Kane, R. T., Thornton, J. A., & Andrews, W. P. (2015). The role of deliberate practice in the development of highly effective psychotherapists. *Psychotherapy, 52*(3), 337–345. https://doi.org/10.1037/pst0000015

Duncan, B. L., Hubble, M. A., & Miller, S. D. (1997). *Psychotherapy with 'impossible' cases: The efficient treatment of therapy veterans.* Norton.

Duncan, B. L., Miller, S. D., Wampold, B. E., & Hubble, M. A. (2010). *The heart and soul of change: Delivering what works in therapy* (2nd ed.). American Psychological Association. https://doi.org/10.1037/12075-000

Goldberg, S. B., Babins-Wagner, R., Rousmaniere, T., Berzins, S., Hoyt, W. T., Whipple, J. L., Miller, S. D., & Wampold, B. E. (2016). Creating a climate for therapist improvement: A case study of an agency focused on outcomes and deliberate practice. *Psychotherapy, 53*(3), 367–375. https://doi.org/10.1037/pst0000060

Goldberg, S. B., Rousmaniere, T., Miller, S. D., Whipple, J., Nielsen, S. L., Hoyt, W. T., & Wampold, B. E. (2016). Do psychotherapists improve with time and experience? A longitudinal analysis of outcomes in a clinical setting. *Journal of Counseling Psychology, 63*(1), 1–11. https://doi.org/10.1037/cou0000131

Grencavage, L. M., & Norcross, J. C. (1990). Where are the commonalities among the therapeutic common factors? *Professional Psychology, Research and Practice, 21*(5), 372–378. https://doi.org/10.1037/0735-7028.21.5.372

Hines, M. (1997). Acceptance versus change in behavior: An interview with Neil Jacobson. *The Family Journal, 6*(3), 244–251. https://doi.org/10.1177/1066480798063016

Hipol, L. J., & Deacon, B. J. (2013). Dissemination of evidence-based practices for anxiety disorders in Wyoming: A survey of practicing psychotherapists. *Behavior Modification, 37*(2), 170–188. https://doi.org/10.1177/0145445512458794

Hofmann, S. G., & Barlow, D. H. (2014). Evidence-based psychological interventions and the common factors approach: The beginnings of a rapprochement? *Psychotherapy, 51*(4), 510–513. https://doi.org/10.1037/a0037045

Hubble, M. A., Duncan, B. L., & Miller, S. (Eds.). (1999). *The heart and soul of change: What works in therapy.* American Psychological Association. https://doi.org/10.1037/11132-000

Katz, M., Hilsenroth, M. J., Gold, J. R., Moore, M., Pitman, S. R., Levy, S. R., & Owen, J. (2019). Adherence, flexibility, and outcome in psychodynamic treatment of depression. *Journal of Counseling Psychology, 66*(1), 94–103. https://doi.org/10.1037/cou0000299

Kramer, S. A. (1986). The termination process in open-ended psychotherapy: Guidelines for clinical practice. *Psychotherapy, 23*(4), 526–531. https://doi.org/10.1037/h0085652

Krebs, P., Norcross, J. C., Nicholson, J. M., & Prochaska, J. O. (2018). Stages of change and psychotherapy outcomes: A review and meta-analysis. *Journal of Clinical Psychology, 74*(11), 1964–1979. https://doi.org/10.1002/jclp.22683

Laska, K. M., & Wampold, B. E. (2014). Ten things to remember about common factor theory. *Psychotherapy, 51*(4), 519–524. https://doi.org/10.1037/a0038245

Levitt, H., Butler, M., & Hill, T. (2006). What clients find helpful in psychotherapy: Developing principles for facilitating moment-to-moment change. *Journal of Counseling Psychology, 53*(3), 314–324. https://doi.org/10.1037/0022-0167.53.3.314

Levitt, H. M., Pomerville, A., & Surace, F. I. (2016). A qualitative meta-analysis examining clients' experiences of psychotherapy: A new agenda. *Psychological Bulletin, 142*(8), 801–830. https://doi.org/10.1037/bul0000057

Mendel, W. M. (1963). The existential emphasis in psychiatry. *American Journal of Psychoanalysis, 23*(1), 29–33. https://doi.org/10.1007/BF01888484

Miller, S. D. (2018, November 20). *Aren't you the anti-evidence-based practice guy? My socks. And other crazy questions.* https://www.scottdmiller.com/arent-you-the-anti-evidence-based-practice-guy-my-socks-and-other-crazy-questions/

Miller, S. D., Hubble, M. A., & Chow, D. (2020). *Better results: Using deliberate practice to improve therapeutic effectiveness.* American Psychological Association. https://doi.org/10.1037/0000191-000

Mohr, D. C. (1995). Negative outcome in psychotherapy: A critical review. *Clinical Psychology: Science and Practice, 2*(1), 1–27. https://doi.org/10.1111/j.1468-2850.1995.tb00022.x

Norcross, J. C., Krebs, P. M., & Prochaska, J. O. (2011). Stages of change. In J. C. Norcross (Ed.), *Psychotherapy relationships that work* (2nd ed., pp. 279–300). Oxford University Press. https://doi.org/10.1093/acprof:oso/9780199737208.003.0014

Norcross, J. C., Zimmerman, B. E., Greenberg, R. P., & Swift, J. K. (2017). Do all therapists do that when saying goodbye? A study of commonalities in termination behaviors. *Psychotherapy, 54*(1), 66–75. https://doi.org/10.1037/pst0000097

Orlinsky, D. E., Ronnestad, M. H., & Willutzky, U. (2004). Fifty years of psychotherapy process-outcome research: Continuity and change. In M. J. Lambert (Ed.), *Bergin and Garfield's handbook of psychotherapy and behavior change* (5th ed.). Wiley.

Patterson, C. H. (1985). *The therapeutic relationship: Foundations for an eclectic psychotherapy.* Brooks/Cole.

Proctor, E. K., & Rosen, A. (1983). Structure in therapy: A conceptual analysis. *Psychotherapy, 20*(2), 202–207. https://doi.org/10.1037/h0088491

Sachs, J. S. (1983). Negative factors in brief psychotherapy: An empirical assessment. *Journal of Consulting and Clinical Psychology, 51*(4), 557–564. https://doi.org/10.1037/0022-006X.51.4.557

Saidipour, P. (2021). The precedent of good enough therapy during unprecedented times. *Clinical Social Work Journal, 49*(4), 429–436. https://doi.org/10.1007/s10615-020-00776-7

Scogin, F., Floyd, M., Jamison, C., Ackerson, J., Landreville, P., & Bissonnette, L. (1996). Negative outcomes: What is the evidence on self-administered treatments? *Journal of Consulting and Clinical Psychology, 64*(5), 1086–1089. https://doi.org/10.1037/0022-006X.64.5.1086

Shapiro, F. (Ed.). (2002). *EMDR as an integrative psychotherapy approach: Experts of diverse orientations explore the paradigm prism.* American Psychological Association. https://doi.org/10.1037/10512-000

Stiles, W. B., & Horvath, A. O. (2017). Appropriate responsiveness as a contribution to therapist effects. In L. G. Castonguay & C. E. Hill (Eds.), *How and why are some therapists better than others? Understanding therapist effects* (pp. 71–84). American Psychological Association. https://doi.org/10.1037/0000034-005

Swift, J. K., & Parkin, S. R. (2017). The client as the expert in psychotherapy: What clinicians and researchers can learn about treatment processes and outcomes from psychotherapy clients. *Journal of Clinical Psychology, 73*(11), 1486–1488. https://doi.org/10.1002/jclp.22528

Tracey, T. J. G. (2003). Concept mapping of therapeutic common factors. *Psychotherapy Research, 13*(4), 401–413. https://doi.org/10.1093/ptr/kpg041

Tracey, T. J. G., Wampold, B. E., Lichtenberg, J. W., & Goodyear, R. K. (2014). Expertise in psychotherapy: An elusive goal? *American Psychologist, 69*(3), 218–229. https://doi.org/10.1037/a0035099

van Minnen, A., Hendriks, L., & Olff, M. (2010). When do trauma experts choose exposure therapy for PTSD patients? A controlled study of therapist and patient factors. *Behaviour Research and Therapy, 48*(4), 312–320. https://doi.org/10.1016/j.brat.2009.12.003

Waller, G. (2009). Evidence-based treatment and therapist drift. *Behaviour Research and Therapy, 47*(2), 119–127. https://doi.org/10.1016/j.brat.2008.10.018

Waller, G., & Turner, H. (2016). Therapist drift redux: Why well-meaning clinicians fail to deliver evidence-based therapy, and how to get back on track. *Behaviour Research and Therapy, 77*, 129–137. https://doi.org/10.1016/j.brat.2015.12.005

Wampold, B. E., Flückiger, C., Del Re, A. C., Yulish, N. E., Frost, N. D., Pace, B. T., Goldberg, S. B., Miller, S. D., Baardseth, T. P., Laska, K. M., & Hilsenroth, M. J. (2017). In pursuit of truth: A critical examination of meta-analyses of cognitive behavior therapy. *Psychotherapy Research, 27*(1), 14–32. https://doi.org/10.1080/10503307.2016.1249433

Wampold, B. E., & Imel, Z. E. (2015). *The great psychotherapy debate: The evidence for what makes psychotherapy work* (2nd ed.). Routledge/Taylor & Francis Group. https://doi.org/10.4324/9780203582015

Webb, C. A., Derubeis, R. J., & Barber, J. P. (2010). Therapist adherence/competence and treatment outcome: A meta-analytic review. *Journal of Consulting and Clinical Psychology, 78*(2), 200–211. https://doi.org/10.1037/a0018912

Weisz, J. R., Donenberg, G. R., Han, S. S., & Kauneckis, D. (1995). Child and adolescent psychotherapy outcomes in experiments versus clinics: Why the disparity? *Journal of Abnormal Child Psychology, 23*(1), 83–106. https://doi.org/10.1007/BF01447046

Yalom, I. D. (2017). *Becoming myself: A psychiatrist's memoir*. Basic Books.

Yulish, N. E., Goldberg, S. B., Frost, N. D., Abbas, M., Oleen-Junk, N. A., Kring, M., Chin, M. Y., Raines, C. R., Soma, C. S., & Wampold, B. E. (2017). The importance of problem-focused treatments: A meta-analysis of anxiety treatments. *Psychotherapy, 54*(4), 321–338. https://doi.org/10.1037/pst0000144

8

Habits

The Key to a Sustainable System of Deliberate Practice

Sam Malins, Scott D. Miller, Mark A. Hubble, and Daryl Chow

We are what we repeatedly do. Excellence, then, is not an act, but a habit.
—WILL DURANT, *THE STORY OF PHILOSOPHY*

DECISION POINT

Begin here if you have read the book *Better Results* (*BR*) and

- are routinely measuring your performance *and*
- have collected sufficient data to establish a reliable, evidence-based profile of your therapeutic effectiveness *and*
- have completed the Taxonomy of Deliberate Practice Activities in Psychotherapy *and*
- have identified an individualized learning objective with the greatest chance of improving your effectiveness *and*
- need help developing consistent deliberate practice routines.

The previous chapters have summarized key factors worthy of deliberate practice (DP) and offered concrete exercises to support the development of related skills. It is hoped the information presented thus far serves to support a decision to employ DP and provide clear direction on what to do. If this has happened, there is some important news: Deciding to engage in DP is half the

---

https://doi.org/10.1037/0000358-009
The Field Guide to Better Results: Evidence-Based Exercises to Improve Therapeutic Effectiveness,
S. D. Miller, D. Chow, S. Malins, and M. A. Hubble (Editors)

battle in becoming more effective. Establishing a system to support implementation and make it a routine is the next step in ensuring DP has a lasting impact (Carden & Wood, 2018).

As has been said before, DP is a long game. Frequently, gains are not noticeable in the short term (Ericsson, 2009; Ericsson et al., 1993). For this reason, reliance on intention, willpower, or motivation is risky and unlikely to be sufficient to sustain engagement following the burst of activity often associated with interest in a new endeavor (Ajzen et al., 2009). Incidentally, brain systems focused on thinking, decision making, and intentions operate differently from those fueling long-standing behavior patterns, which are much slower to change and require less conscious decision making (Wood & Rünger, 2016). Said another way, force of will may be sufficient to scale a mountain today but not support a daily exercise regimen committed to yesterday. Doing the latter requires establishing a new *habit*—defined as "a settled tendency or usual manner of behavior . . . that has become nearly or completely involuntary" (Merriam-Webster, n.d.). Thankfully, research provides a clear picture of the process involved.

This chapter will

- briefly summarize the empirical literature on long-term habit formation,

- identify evidence-based principles for making DP a default part of one's daily routine, and

- provide exercises to support the development of and overcome any barriers to a "DP habit."

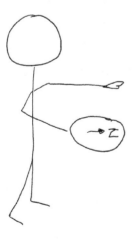

FIELD GUIDE TIP

Set the *Field Guide* down and reread Chapter 14 in *Better Results*, "Designing a Sustainable System of Deliberate Practice."

Next, using a scale from 1 to 5 (where 5 is *high* and 1 *low*), rate how well you have implemented each of the four elements of a successful deliberate practice plan. Known as ARPS, these include (a) automated structure, (b) reference point, (c) playful experimentations, and (d) support persons.

Reading further without first working at improving the implementation of any element scoring 3 or lower risks DP becoming just one more interesting but unused idea a therapist will come across in the course of their professional lifetime (Michie et al., 2009; Webb & Sheeran, 2006).

REVIEW OF THE RESEARCH

A defining characteristic of a habit is that it occurs with little conscious effort or thought (Mazar & Wood, 2018; Verplanken, 2006; Wood & Neal, 2007). Central to its development is "automaticity," wherein environmental cues trigger the execution of a predictable pattern of behavior outside a person's intention or awareness (Bargh, 1994). This definition clarifies habit formation is more than repetition (although, as will be seen, doing something over and again plays a role) or merely the development of a sense of familiarity. Speaking metaphorically, an established habit is like part of the furniture. It exists and is employed effectively, with neither acknowledgment nor attention.

Wood (2019) identified three reliable pathways to habit formation and revision. The first is regular repetition. While it is widely believed habits take 21 days to form, the evidence shows otherwise. It takes much longer. In what is now known as the seminal study on the subject, Lally et al. (2010) asked 96 volunteers to work on developing a new, healthy habit (e.g., eating, drinking, or activity). Data on the frequency of completion and degree of automaticity indicated an average of 66 days were required (with a range from 18 to 254), with more complex changes taking longer. Several other findings from the study are informative. First, missing the occasional opportunity to practice a new behavior resulted in only a negligible drop in the development of automaticity. Clearly, hope for success is not dashed when choice or circumstance results in a "time-out." Second, context is important (Lally et al., 2011). Practicing in the same location on the same day at the same time is facilitative. Environments with unique or memorable features are also helpful, providing cues for action (e.g., "I do 20 minutes DP every Friday in my office following the team meeting, and that's also when I have a caramel latte each week"). Third, and finally, the wide range in times reported by Lally and colleagues indicates some habits can form much more quickly. Identifying these and breaking down more complex ones into their smaller constituent parts makes shorter, easier-to-schedule practice periods possible, thereby increasing opportunities for automation to develop more quickly (Kaushal & Rhodes, 2015). While on the subject of time, Fogg (2020), following years of research at the Behavior Design Lab at Stanford, concluded consistency is far more important than amount. Doing a few minutes of a given activity on a regular basis, he reported, yields more dividends than regularly increasing the time allotted to practice. The reason is simple. It is easier to commit to and follow through with small "entry points," recognizing they can always be extended. By contrast, setting up longer periods and then failing to fill the time with practice can sponsor frustration and disappointment.

The second pathway is rewards. Forming new habits requires persistence despite the pressure of distractions or more desirable pursuits (Andersson & Bergman, 2011). Along the way, rewards can help maintain focus and concentration, with particular types superior to others. Intrinsic rewards (e.g., reminders of internal motivations) tend to be more effective than extrinsic (e.g., money, validation by managers or a supervisor; Lally & Gardner, 2013).

External rewards *can* enhance habit formation, provided they do not become the sole purpose of practicing (Deci et al., 1999). For example, a meta-analysis of 40 years of research conducted by Cerasoli et al. (2014) found extrinsic rewards negatively alter the link between internal motivation and performance outcomes. In particular, when the locus of control shifts to someone or something outside the self, what one once did because it felt right or good becomes a chore.

The last pathway is reducing friction. Consider the following: slightly delaying the time an elevator takes to arrive once the call button is pressed, increasing the distance one must cross to access unhealthy food, and placing recycling bins close to workers. All share a common characteristic. They either increase or decrease the likelihood of a desirable behavior occurring and being repeated: increasing the use of stairs, decreasing the consumption of "junk" food, and separating reusables from trash, respectively (Clohessy et al., 2019; Houten et al., 1981; Ludwig et al., 1998; Rozin et al., 2011; Soler et al., 2010; Wansink et al., 2016). In the literature, such elements or conditions have come to be called "friction" (Wood & Neal, 2016). Common to all work environments and pursuits, they can be modified in the service of promoting habit formation. Reduce the source to increase behavioral options and repetition; increase them, and the opposite occurs.

In their study of highly effective therapists, Miller and Hubble (2011) found those who eventually rise to the top, becoming "supershrinks," do not "exist in a vacuum, bursting suddenly on the scene following years of private toil" (p. 25). Far from it. The best reside in a social context consisting of people—family, partners, colleagues, supervisors, teachers, coaches—who nurture and support habits of excellence. It is familiar to anyone committed to DP: What is required is continuously reaching for performance objectives beyond one's current ability, adopting an error-centric mindset (i.e., welcoming mistakes as learning opportunities), and being open to feedback.

Greaney et al. (2018) reported on the role of social support in changing risky habits (e.g., smoking, unhealthy eating, sedentary lifestyle). Participants who identified one supportive person were significantly more successful than those who tried to go it alone. "Participants identifying multiple support persons," the authors found, "had 100% greater reduction" in multiple risky behaviors (p. 198). Thus, when it comes to developing new habits, social support is good, and more is better.

EVIDENCE-BASED PRINCIPLES RELATED TO HABIT FORMATION

No doubt, DP has the potential to help you achieve better results. The same is seen in many domains of human performance. The challenge, once you begin to implement it, is sustainability. Detailed suggestions were provided in Chapter 14 of *Better Results* (*BR*; pp. 157–170). If you haven't already done so and find yourself struggling to be consistent, we recommend returning to that section first, paying particular attention to the discussion of ARPS (automated structure, reference point, playful experimentations, and support persons). For ease of reference, Table 14.2 from *BR* summarizing the four elements and potential action steps is represented here.

System	Think . . .	Description
Automated structure	Algorithmically	Schedule it
		Protect the DP environment
		Create a black box
Reference point	Directionally	Keep one eye on your outcome data
		Keep the other eye on your current learning objectives (see TDPA)
Playful experimentation	Like a child	Lateral learning
		Call on your ideal identity
		The "it's never too late to have a good session" technique
		Arrange a surprise party
		Test to learn, don't learn for the test
Support	Communally	Form a scenius community
		Seek out separate coaches for performance and development

The ARPS framework is supported by the research on habit formation reviewed in this chapter. By definition, habits do not require planning or forethought. Transforming new behaviors into habits does, however. You must establish systems (e.g., turning off the phone, email notifications) and structures (e.g., time, place, focus) that make engagement in DP *automatic*, independent of one's motivational state. Rewards are also important. Here is where having a *reference point* is essential. What better reward for DP exists than comparing your current performance data with your baseline and seeing progress, the results of your hard work? In addition, maintaining a *playful* attitude and spirit of *experimentation*—especially in the face of the setbacks and mistakes that are an integral part of DP—supports the risk-taking necessary for the development of new ways of thinking and behaving (Brown & Vaughan, 2009). Last but not least is social support; its importance cannot be overstated. Friends, colleagues, coaches, and a community greatly increase the chances of successful habit formation.

In addition to ARPS, three principles emerge from the review of the empirical literature.

Principle 1: Identity Matters

The role therapist identity can play in developing and sustaining DP habits was introduced, along with concrete exercises, in *BR* (Miller et al., 2020, pp. 123–137, 165). Simply put, our professional identity reflects the values we hold about the world and our work. When consciously and intentionally aligned with our DP objectives, the time and effort we devote to improving our ability to help become intrinsically rewarding, adding meaning and purpose to our engagement in challenging, long-term projects. Such alignment, research further shows, enhances our sense of personal authenticity (Gan & Chen, 2017).

Principle 2: Anticipation Is the Best Defense

Having a clear DP plan helps in habit formation. That said, many are too idealistic in scope, failing to consider the barriers likely encountered along the way (Buehler et al., 2010). When it comes to goal setting, current evidence suggests the combination of two strategies works best: first, visualizing the desired objective (e.g., reviewing outcome data twice a week, spending 20 minutes twice a week at the end of the workday completing one of the many exercises recommended in the *Field Guide*) and, second, connecting it with the key barriers to achievement and concrete plans for addressing such obstacles. Making it easy to anticipate and adapt to problems encountered (i.e., if situation X arises, I will use strategy Y to achieve goal Z) lessens the chance of disrupting automaticity, characteristic of established habits (Gollwitzer, 1999).

Principle 3: You Have Done This Before

More than 40% of what we do on a daily basis is habitual—patterns of thinking and behaving you have already successfully created (Wood, 2019). Whether deemed "good" or "bad," "healthy," or "unhealthy," the same process is involved. In short, you have done this before. Habits may be hard work to establish or change, but doing so is nothing new. Using what you have learned from these experiences will be helpful in developing the habits necessary to sustain your engagement in DP.

EXERCISES FOR DEVELOPING THE HABITS SUPPORTING DELIBERATE PRACTICE

The following exercises are aligned with the principles and aim to help make DP a permanent *and* evolving part of your professional development. Each is to be completed within a specified time—most within 5 minutes. For this reason, it will be helpful to have a timer present. No need for a fancy stopwatch because most mobile phones come with one. Each can be completed alone or together with a colleague or coach. Table 8.1 provides an at-a-glance summary of the principles and their associated exercises. The first four revisit the ARPS framework.

TABLE 8.1. Summary of Principles and Exercises

Principle	Principle summary	Related exercises	Exercise summary
1: Automated structure	Build DP into your existing automated habits.	1: Make it so	Schedule DP and specify the particular activities for each episode to make them more likely to happen.
		2: Make it easy and rewarding	Incorporate small, but meaningful rewards into DP, ideally linked to its overall purpose.
2: Reference point	Finding a range of ways to track progress toward goals helps when improvement is slow.	3: Where are you now?	Build qualitative and quantitative performance benchmarks into DP alongside regular reviews.
3: Playful experimentation	Approach DP with playfulness to maintain creativity and manage difficulties.	4: Playful progress	Use comic rewards, light-hearted exercises with friends and family, music or rhyming in DP.
		5: All change	Capitalize on current or upcoming changes that disrupt existing habits and may make room for new ones.
		6: Parallel play	Try out DP in areas of your life other than psychotherapy, particularly active rest hobbies.
4: Support	Do not approach DP alone; invite and recruit others to support DP.	7: Choosing a coach	Identify one or two potential coaches and contact them for an initial conversation.
		8: Building a support network	Reach out to a peer or network of peers who are either using DP or you think could benefit from trying it.
5: Identify your identity	Build rewards into DP that remind you of who you are becoming as you practice.	9: The retirement party	Write a speech that includes what you would like to be said about you and your future work at retirement.
6: Forewarned is forearmed	When planning goals, make sure they account for the most important barriers to progress.	10: The premortem	Plan for potential problems with implementing DP by imagining you have already failed and why it happened.
7: You have done this before	Use strategies and knowledge you have gained from building habits previously.	11: This is not your first rodeo	Go through your habit history, identifying factors that helped and hindered you in building habits.

Note. DP = deliberate practice.

Exercise 1: Make It So (5 minutes)

Principle: The *A* in ARPS
Purpose

Busyness is a common barrier to making DP routine. Scheduling ahead of time is the "antidote." Start small—10 to 20 minutes. Eliminate as much prep work as possible by identifying specific tasks you can begin at the outset of your scheduled time. Small, meaningful, and clearly defined tasks will help you to get going and make the time feel like it was well spent, especially at the start.

Task

Make short periods of DP a part of your schedule for the coming month. To ensure success,

- make it obvious in your calendar so it cannot be overwritten and is visible to you and anyone who handles your schedule;
- connect your DP to an established habit in your work routine (e.g., after lunch or a regular meeting that is unlikely to be canceled);
- reward yourself after completing a DP activity;
- include time to rest in the scheduling—DP is effortful, so shorter, intensive periods of DP followed by brief rests is more effective; and
- share what you are doing with others, friends, family, and particularly colleagues who are incorporating DP in their work.

Exercise 2: Make It Easy and Rewarding (5–15 minutes)

Principle: 1
Purpose

It is learning theory 101. What you reward increases. Punishment suppresses behavior. Identifying small, meaningful rewards will support your motivation to continue DP, especially at the outset when the most effort is required.

Task

Mindful of the research reviewed earlier documenting the potency of intrinsic rewards and the reduction of friction in habit formation, devote time to creating a work environment that makes DP easy, enjoyable, and productive (people, decor, artwork, furniture, natural light, everyday conveniences, and tangible rewards).

- Make a list of your reasons for doing DP. In constructing or organizing your workspace, find ways to remind yourself of your best intentions. It could be a picture, an objet d'art, a poster with an inspirational quote, or an avatar on your social media profile. It could even be a reminder on your phone or computer.

- Spend a few minutes each week for 1 month noting what gets in the way of your DP. It could be clutter, excessive noise, hunger, size of caseload, or anything. The following month, rank order the barriers from most to least disruptive and start addressing them one at a time, starting at the top.

- Make a list of people with whom you will share your successes and struggles, seeking out cheerleaders rather than naysayers, team players rather than competitors.

Exercise 3: Where Are You Now? (5–15 minutes)

Principle: 2
Purpose
In a long-term learning project such as DP, having a regular, understandable assessment of key performance indicators helps identify progress where it might not be noticed otherwise.

Task
Identify and/or build in key performance reference points of where you are now:

- Find out or calculate your current outcome performance metrics, ideally benchmarked against the performance of other psychotherapists, as discussed in Chapter 1.

- Identify your current individualized learning objective, preferably using recordings of your sessions to help you discover it, coupled with your aggregated outcomes.

- Keep a recording of a recent session that highlighted some current skill deficits you will work on with DP, where you have permission to retain the recording for a few months. Diarize a time to listen back to this session segment after a couple of months of DP.

- Use your current "how I do therapy" blueprint (see Chapter 1 for further explanation) as a qualitative benchmark, redrafting and reviewing it as your practice evolves with DP.

At least once a month, review these way markers as part of your DP to help identify points of change.

Exercise 4: Playful Progress (5–15 minutes)

Principle: 3
Purpose
DP can be hard, and the slow progress can be disheartening. Therefore, this exercise aims to help find ways of bringing playfulness to the process, which can maintain a sense of fun, creativity, and lightheartedness.

Task

Brainstorm ways to bring playfulness into DP, then try one or two out at your next DP sessions. Some examples of bringing playfulness to DP are

- setting your individualized learning goals to music, such as a jingle on a commercial (alternatively, work out a rhyme that describes your learning objective);

- trying out the therapeutic skills you are developing in DP with friends and family members during casual conversations and seeking their feedback in a lighthearted way; and

- making comic rewards for attempts at improvement (e.g., winning a jelly bean or chocolate, gaining a plastic trophy for a set number of DP hours).

Exercise 5: All Change (5–15 minutes)

Principle: 3
Purpose
This exercise aims to help you identify areas of upcoming or existing change that may present a way to playfully introduce new habits that could support DP.

Task
Take 2 to 5 minutes to list changes that are going on in your home or work life at the moment or that have occurred recently. Your list can include anything, but the following are some examples to prompt your thinking to include changes you may have badged as positive or negative:

- changing jobs (Yes. Drastic. But some jobs are hazardous to your well-being and are not conducive to your development.)
- moving desks
- working in a new way or system
- having a new supervisor or coach
- getting a new pet, child, or partner

Consider the following:

- How could these changes disrupt the status quo in a way that paves a route to new DP-related habits? Take 2 to 5 minutes to brainstorm ways that changes in your life might facilitate the introduction of DP.

- Take 1 to 5 minutes to consider where you might start with leveraging this change to support DP.

Exercise 6: Parallel Play (5–10 minutes to start)

Principle: 3
Purpose
Many high achievers in demanding roles find *active rest*, hobbies that, in some ways, reflect themes of their work but without key drawbacks. A quintessential

example of this is academics who are rock climbers: Climbing takes thought, planning, and a strategy and is time consuming—just like research. However, with rock climbing, you get the exhilaration of success by the end of the day rather than having to wait months or years for the outcome of research (Mitchell, 1983). This exercise aims to identify activities that are outside the realm of psychotherapy DP but might draw on parallel principles.

Task

Are there any activities you do or used to do that can give a similar sense of achievement or satisfaction as psychotherapy but in a different sphere of life? For example, playing basketball may, at face value, look completely unrelated to psychotherapy, but perhaps there are parallels in the way that you aim to collaborate with players on your team or the way you strategically analyze how to address particularly challenging defenses in a time-out. However, basketball also avoids some of the difficulties of psychotherapy—you get to know how it pans out by the end of the evening rather than working for several weeks, months, or years to see the fruit of your labor.

- Identify an activity or hobby that is like psychotherapy but not psychotherapy, and consider trying DP in this area at the same time as DP in psychotherapy. Continuing our basketball example, rather than just shooting around at random when you are starting to play, work out a short practice that is likely to help you shoot more effectively, even though it may take small incremental gains. A similar approach could be taken to swimming, running, chess, crochet, or any hobby requiring specific trainable skills. Think of a way of doing DP that isn't psychotherapy DP and can be playful or fun.

- If you once found an activity that gave similar satisfaction to psychotherapy, but you no longer do it, now might be a good time to restart this pursuit to provide a release from the efforts of DP for psychotherapy in a different area that could provide a similar sense of reward.

Exercise 7: Choosing a Coach (5–10 minutes)

Principle: 4

Purpose

Given the central role of a coach in DP, this exercise aims to help identify someone with the appropriate characteristics.

Task

Identify one or two potential coaches and contact them one at a time for an initial conversation. Aim high with this choice (see *BR*; Miller et al., 2020, pp. 35–39, 112–113). Aim for someone who you feel

- has authority but is not authoritarian,
- is invested in you finding your best way of doing things rather than replicating their approach,

- is clear about where you want help, and
- has sufficient skill to be able to identify your deficits and offer strategies to remediate them.

Exercise 8: Building a Support Network (5–10 minutes)

Principle: 4
Purpose

Given the central role of a coach in DP, this exercise aims to help identify someone with the appropriate characteristics.

Task

Reach out to a peer or network of peers who are embarking on the use of DP in their practice or people you would like to encourage to do so. You could collaborate with someone who works in your area or reach out beyond. The International Center for Clinical Excellence network might be a useful starting place (see https://www.iccexcellence.com).

Exercise 9: The Retirement Party (30 minutes)

Principle: 5
Purpose

This is an adaptation of an existing exercise (Harris, 2009) that aims to link personal values with DP and the longer term results of persisting with it.

Task

Imagine you set up a sustainable system of DP from this day forth. It is now your retirement party, and a close friend who knows you well and cares about you gets up in front of your family, friends, and colleagues to give a speech about how you conducted the remainder of your career. What would you want them to be able to say about you and what was important to you during the rest of your career?

- Take a couple of minutes to picture the scene and imagine what principles or values you would like to hear your friend say that you upheld and stood for through the rest of your career. Write these down (5 minutes).

- Now your friend describes some of the things you did on a regular basis that showed what you valued. What routine practices would you like them to be able to cite? Some might be activities you already do, but some may be activities you aspire to do. List these regular, routine activities (3 minutes).

- Where would DP fit in this speech? What would your friend say about
  - what you did,
  - how you made DP part of your day-to-day life,
  - how you overcame barriers to keep it going throughout your career, and
  - how DP impacted your personal and professional life and those you encountered?

- Spend 3 minutes on each of these areas, writing down what you would like your friend to be able to say at your retirement party.

- Look back over what you have written either alone, with a colleague who has completed the same exercise or with a coach or supervisor. Spend 10 minutes reviewing these questions in reflection on this exercise:
  - What are the central threads running throughout the speech that are components of your identity you would like to nurture and grow?
  - How might DP support this?
  - What does this exercise tell you about how DP might need to look for it to play a consistent role in your career?
  - What does this speech tell you about where to start with implementing DP now?

Exercise 9: The 5-Minute Version

Imagine a close friend giving a speech about the rest of your career at your retirement party. Spend a minute each on (a) thinking about where DP would fit in this speech, (b) how DP would support the important values you would like to uphold in the rest of your career, and (c) how DP would look and fit in your ideal future career. Now spend 2 minutes reflecting on what this tells you about how you want DP to affect your identity and where it would be best to start with this system.

Exercise 10: The Premortem (30 minutes)

Principle: 6
Purpose
Prospective hindsight is a process of imagining a future event has already happened and helps people to be more accurate in predicting how plans will progress (Mitchell et al., 1989). Gary Klein (2007) applied this approach to project planning by asking participants to imagine a project has already failed. This approach helped participants identify weaknesses in the plan and adjustments required to improve it. The premortem approach is applied to DP implementation in this exercise.

Task
Imagine you started a system of DP today, and you are looking back a year from now. It has been a complete disaster and has failed miserably.

- Write a detailed description of why it failed so badly and all the reasons that caused the failure. Remember to write in the past tense, looking back a year from now. This helps overcome futuristic optimism and the planning fallacy and gives clarity on potential barriers that may be difficult to call to mind when hopeful about a future plan (10 minutes).

- Create an "if–then" guide for each potential problem your DP system may face. Discuss this with a colleague or a coach or supervisor to help brainstorm adaptations to your plans that would account for the barriers you are likely to face (15 minutes).

- In case these were not identified in your premortem, some of the most likely barriers are described next. Spend 5 minutes checking whether the plans you have made will address these issues:
  - **The pull to perform:** It is unlikely anyone in your service will be pushing you to make DP happen, but there may well be a pull to get more clients seen more quickly, which could cut into DP time. How would you deal with that?
  - **A hard day's night:** As described earlier, DP is effortful and tiring, so it may not be the most appetizing activity to follow a hard day, week, or therapy session. The mental effort involved in DP could spoil your plans when internal resources are depleted. How could you overcome that?
  - **Resource restriction:** Professional development activities are limited in almost all psychotherapy organizations and are usually focused on attaining competence (or at least familiarity) with new therapeutic techniques. This is unlikely to leave much room for DP, which aims to be an ongoing component of professional development for all therapy techniques. How would you tackle this conundrum?
  - **Softening the blow (maybe too much):** Some supervisors or coaches might feel DP is a way of being excessively self-critical. They may emphasize the complexity of a client's problems, say that your efforts are good enough, or perhaps infer that you are nit-picking by identifying a small unhelpful habit in the grand scheme of things. In general, your support systems may aim to comfort you in a well-meaning manner when you identify microskills for DP. There may be truth in what they say, but how will you manage this dynamic to progress with DP?

Exercise 10: The 5-Minute Version

Spend 2 minutes imagining that your attempt to embed DP fails terribly over the coming months. Spend 1 minute identifying the top three reasons why this happened. Pick the most important of these three reasons and take 2 minutes to make at least one "if–then" plan for how you would tackle it.

Exercise 11a: This Is Not Your First Rodeo, Part 1—Your Forgotten Rodeos (15–20 minutes for each part, ideally alone initially, then reflect with a coach, practice partner, or small group)

Principle: 7
Purpose
This series of exercises aims to draw on your previous experience of building sustainable habits (or attempts to do so) and how this can inform your plan for a sustainable DP system.

Task

Think through times in your personal or professional life when you have felt excited, enthused, determined, or energized to try something new or different, and it has not worked out. Perhaps you started but could not stick with it, or nothing happened at all. With the benefit of hindsight, what got in the way in each of these areas?

- **Existing routine:** Specifically, what daily structures or habits prevented this from becoming part of your normal life?

- **Environment:** What environmental cues (or the absence of such cues) might have made it harder for this habit to form?

- **People:** Which people did you not have on board who might have helped with this (or potentially obstructed habit formation because they were not involved)?

- **Willpower:** How much importance did you place on willpower in making this habit work?

Exercise 11b: This Is Not Your First Rodeo, Part 2—Your Winning Rodeos (15–20 minutes)

Principle: 7

Purpose

This part of the exercise aims to make use of helpful strategies established in previous or existing habits that may be applied to DP.

Task

Think about helpful, healthy, and/or valued activities you do regularly as part of your current routine at work or in your personal life.

- Specifically identify two to five habits or routines that are important to you that support aspects of your work or your life more broadly. These are likely to be habits you take completely for granted and may be so deep in the water that you could easily overlook them. If it is hard to think of these, go through a typical day from waking up, and in 30-minute intervals, identify activities that are helpful for you.

- What helped these habits to form? Again, be aware of the urge just to shrug your shoulders and say, "Well, they just seemed to happen." If this is your experience, it is just underlining that massive, long-standing bouts of willpower are not the key to long-standing habit formation. This is the beauty of habits: Their ability to continue is barely noticeable in terms of conscious effort, but this makes it difficult to identify their mechanisms. One way to do this is to track back to a time when you were not doing the habit and consider how it started.

- Think through the role played by each of the following areas in forming each habit.

  - **Existing routine:** What aspects of your existing routine (at the time the habit was started) helped the new habit to form? In what way did existing behaviors cue the new habit? What factors were reinforcing, rewarding, reminding, or recognizing occasions of carrying out the habit?

  - **Environment:** What was going on in your environment that cued the new habit—even if in small, seemingly trivial ways, such as objects being close and accessible or far away and inaccessible?

  - **People:** Who was involved in either helping form this habit (maybe you did it with someone or for someone) or supported you in forming this habit? What did they do? How did you get them involved?

  - **Willpower:** In the long term, what role did willpower play in establishing this habit?

Exercise 11c: This Is Not Your First Rodeo, Part 3—Your Next Rodeo (15–20 minutes)

Principle: 7
Purpose
The final part of this exercise uses what was learned in Parts 1 and 2 to distill strategies likely to be helpful in DP, alongside possible barriers and how to manage them.

Task
Reflect on the key themes you noticed while completing Parts 1 and 2 with a coach, practice partner, or small group who have also completed the exercise.

- Use your reflections from Parts 1 and 2 to complete Table 8.2.

- Identify what has been helpful and unhelpful from your previous experiences of successful and unsuccessful attempts to integrate new habits into your routine.

TABLE 8.2. Applying Learning From Previous Habits to a Sustainable System of DP

Areas for rewards, reinforcers, reminders, and recognition	Unhelpful with habits before	Helpful with habits before	Helpful for DP habits now
Integrating into routine			
Environmental cues			
Involvement of people			
Where willpower fits			

- From these elements, what do you think might help you establish a sustainable system of DP? Pay particular attention to rewards, reinforcers, reminders, and recognition in the way you could
  - integrate DP into your existing routine,
  - shape your environment to encourage DP,
  - helpfully involve other people in your DP habits, and
  - keep willpower in its rightful place.

Exercise 11: The 5-Minute Version

Spend 2 minutes identifying healthy, helpful, and/or valued activities you carry out on a regular basis. Now spend 2 minutes identifying habits you wanted to form but failed to do so. Take a minute to reflect on the differences between the two and how this informs your approach to embedding DP sustainably.

SUMMARY

No matter how motivated you feel about DP right now or how strong you perceive your willpower to be, the main message of this chapter is that the structured systems you build around DP hold more sway in keeping you going in the longer term. Specifically, this chapter outlined current evidence on using rewards linked to intrinsic motivators, managing the environment to promote and protect DP, finding appropriate support, and tracking progress. Perhaps most important, this chapter discussed the likelihood of failure and how responses to obstacles can be key in the continuation of a challenging but important activity like DP. Like some sustainable practices in energy use, the activities recommended in this chapter could seem to slow immediate progress and feel costly, but in the long run, aim to generate their own energy, requiring less motivation-related resources over time for sustaining DP.

FURTHER READINGS AND RESOURCES

This chapter reviewed the available research, identified evidence-based principles, and suggested a DP practice plan. Additional research and recommendations can be found in the following:

Clear, J. (2018). *Atomic habits: An easy and proven way to build good habits and break bad ones*. Random House.
   This book offers a simple and practical explanation of how habits are formed and how the mechanisms for habit formation can be harnessed strategically.

Ericsson, K. A., & Pool, R. (2016). *Peak: Secrets from the science of expertise*. Houghton Mifflin Harcourt.
   A summary of the evidence on DP and its processes and outcomes, alongside the experience of using it.

Gardner, B., Abraham, C., Lally, P., & de Bruijn, G. J. (2012). Towards parsimony in habit measurement: Testing the convergent and predictive validity of an automaticity subscale of the Self-Report Habit Index. *International Journal of Behavioral Nutrition and Physical Activity, 9*(1), 1–12. https://doi.org/10.1186/1479-5868-9-102.
A brief self-report assessment of whether automaticity has been achieved.

Miller, S. D., Hubble, M. A., & Chow, D. (2020). *Better results: Using deliberate practice to improve therapeutic effectiveness.* American Psychological Association. https://doi.org/10.1037/0000191-000
An explanation of how DP can be applied to psychotherapy to improve outcomes.

Pang, A. S. K. (2016). *Rest: Why you get more done when you work less.* Basic Books.
A deep dive into case studies and more generalizable evidence on the value of rest for effective and mentally taxing work.

Wood, W. (2019). *Good habits, bad habits: The science of making positive changes that stick.* Macmillan.
An explanation of the science behind habit formation from a leading researcher in the field.

REFERENCES

Ajzen, I., Czasch, C., & Flood, M. G. (2009). From intentions to behavior: Implementation intention, commitment, and conscientiousness. *Journal of Applied Social Psychology, 39*(6), 1356–1372. https://doi.org/10.1111/j.1559-1816.2009.00485.x

Andersson, H., & Bergman, L. R. (2011). The role of task persistence in young adolescence for successful educational and occupational attainment in middle adulthood. *Developmental Psychology, 47*(4), 950–960. https://doi.org/10.1037/a0023786

Bargh, J. A. (1994). The four horsemen of automaticity: Awareness, intention, efficiency, and control in social cognition. In R. S. Wyer & T. K. Srull (Eds.), *Handbook of social cognition: Vol 1. Basic processes* (pp. 1–40). Erlbaum.

Brown, S., & Vaughan, C. (2009). *Play: How it shapes the brain, opens the imagination, and invigorates the soul.* Penguin.

Buehler, R., Griffin, D., & Peetz, J. (2010). The planning fallacy: Cognitive, motivational, and social origins. In M. P. Zanna & J. M. Olson (Eds.), *Advances in experimental social psychology* (Vol. 43, pp. 1–62). Academic Press. https://doi.org/10.1016/S0065-2601(10)43001-4

Carden, L., & Wood, W. (2018). Habit formation and change. *Current Opinion in Behavioral Sciences, 20,* 117–122. https://doi.org/10.1016/j.cobeha.2017.12.009

Cerasoli, C. P., Nicklin, J. M., & Ford, M. T. (2014). Intrinsic motivation and extrinsic incentives jointly predict performance: A 40-year meta-analysis. *Psychological Bulletin, 140*(4), 980–1008. https://doi.org/10.1037/a0035661

Clohessy, S., Walasek, L., & Meyer, C. (2019). Factors influencing employees' eating behaviours in the office-based workplace: A systematic review. *Obesity Reviews, 20*(12), 1771–1780. https://doi.org/10.1111/obr.12920

Deci, E. L., Koestner, R., & Ryan, R. M. (1999). The undermining effect is a reality after all—Extrinsic rewards, task interest, and self-determination: Reply to Eisenberger, Pierce, and Cameron (1999) and Lepper, Henderlong, and Gingras (1999). *Psychological Bulletin, 125*(6), 692–700. https://doi.org/10.1037/0033-2909.125.6.692

Ericsson, K. A. (2009). Enhancing the development of professional performance: Implications from the study of deliberate practice. In K. A. Ericsson (Ed.), *Development of professional expertise: Toward measurement of expert performance and design of optimal learning environments* (pp. 405–431). Cambridge University Press. https://doi.org/10.1017/CBO9780511609817

Ericsson, K. A., Krampe, R. T., & Tesch-Römer, C. (1993). The role of deliberate practice in the acquisition of expert performance. *Psychological Review, 100*(3), 363–406. https://doi.org/10.1037/0033-295X.100.3.363

Fogg, B. (2020). *Tiny habits: The small changes that change everything.* Houghton Mifflin Harcourt.

Gan, M., & Chen, S. (2017). Being your actual or ideal self? What it means to feel authentic in a relationship. *Personality and Social Psychology Bulletin, 43*(4), 465–478. https://doi.org/10.1177/0146167216688211

Gollwitzer, P. M. (1999). Implementation intentions: Strong effects of simple plans. *American Psychologist, 54*(7), 493–503. https://doi.org/10.1037/0003-066X.54.7.493

Greaney, M. L., Puleo, E., Sprunck-Harrild, K., Haines, J., Houghton, S. C., & Emmons, K. M. (2018). Social support for changing multiple behaviors: Factors associated with seeking support and the impact of offered support. *Health Education & Behavior, 45*(2), 198–206. https://doi.org/10.1177/1090198117712333

Harris, R. (2009). *ACT made simple.* New Harbinger.

Houten, R. V., Nau, P. A., & Merrigan, M. (1981). Reducing elevator energy use: A comparison of posted feedback and reduced elevator convenience. *Journal of Applied Behavior Analysis, 14*(4), 377–387. https://doi.org/10.1901/jaba.1981.14-377

Kaushal, N., & Rhodes, R. E. (2015). Exercise habit formation in new gym members: A longitudinal study. *Journal of Behavioral Medicine, 38*(4), 652–663. https://doi.org/10.1007/s10865-015-9640-7

Klein, G. (2007). Performing a premortem. *Harvard Business Review, 85*(9), 18–19.

Lally, P., & Gardner, B. (2013). Promoting habit formation. *Health Psychology Review, 7*(Suppl. 1), S137–S158. https://doi.org/10.1080/17437199.2011.603640

Lally, P., Van Jaarsveld, C. H., Potts, H. W., & Wardle, J. (2010). How are habits formed: Modelling habit formation in the real world. *European Journal of Social Psychology, 40*(6), 998–1009. https://doi.org/10.1002/ejsp.674

Lally, P., Wardle, J., & Gardner, B. (2011). Experiences of habit formation: A qualitative study. *Psychology, Health & Medicine, 16*(4), 484–489. https://doi.org/10.1080/13548506.2011.555774

Ludwig, T. D., Gray, T. W., & Rowell, A. (1998). Increasing recycling in academic buildings: A systematic replication. *Journal of Applied Behavior Analysis, 31*(4), 683–686. https://doi.org/10.1901/jaba.1998.31-683

Mazar, A., & Wood, W. (2018). Defining habit in psychology. In B. Verplanken (Ed.), *The psychology of habit* (pp. 13–29). Springer International. https://doi.org/10.1007/978-3-319-97529-0_2

Merriam-Webster. (n.d.). Habit. In *Merriam-Webster.com dictionary.* Retrieved December 13, 2022, from https://www.merriam-webster.com/dictionary/habit

Michie, S., Abraham, C., Whittington, C., McAteer, J., & Gupta, S. (2009). Effective techniques in healthy eating and physical activity interventions: A meta-regression. *Health Psychology, 28*(6), 690–701. https://doi.org/10.1037/a0016136

Miller, S. D., & Hubble, M. A. (2011). The road to mastery. *Psychotherapy Networker, 35*(3), 22–31.

Miller, S. D., Hubble, M. A., & Chow, D. (2020). *Better results: Using deliberate practice to improve therapeutic effectiveness.* American Psychological Association. https://doi.org/10.1037/0000191-000

Mitchell, D. J., Edward Russo, J., & Pennington, N. (1989). Back to the future: Temporal perspective in the explanation of events. *Journal of Behavioral Decision Making, 2*(1), 25–38. https://doi.org/10.1002/bdm.3960020103

Mitchell, R. G. (1983). *Mountain experience: The psychology and sociology of adventure.* University of Chicago Press.

Rozin, P., Scott, S. E., Dingley, M., Urbanek, J. K., Jiang, H., & Kaltenbach, M. (2011). Nudge to nobesity I: Minor changes in accessibility decrease food intake. *Judgment and Decision Making, 6*(4), 323–332.

Soler, R. E., Leeks, K. D., Buchanan, L. R., Brownson, R. C., Heath, G. W., Hopkins, D. H., & the Task Force on Community Preventive Services. (2010). Point-of-decision prompts to increase stair use. A systematic review update. *American Journal of Preventive Medicine, 38*(2, Suppl), S292–S300. https://doi.org/10.1016/j.amepre.2009.10.028

Verplanken, B. (2006). Beyond frequency: Habit as mental construct. *British Journal of Social Psychology, 45*(3), 639–656. https://doi.org/10.1348/014466605X49122

Wansink, B., Hanks, A. S., & Kaipainen, K. (2016). Slim by design: Kitchen counter correlates of obesity. *Health Education & Behavior, 43*(5), 552–558. https://doi.org/10.1177/1090198115610571

Webb, T. L., & Sheeran, P. (2006). Does changing behavioral intentions engender behavior change? A meta-analysis of the experimental evidence. *Psychological Bulletin, 132*(2), 249–268. https://doi.org/10.1037/0033-2909.132.2.249

Wood, W. (2019). *Good habits, bad habits: The science of making positive changes that stick.* Pan Books.

Wood, W., & Neal, D. T. (2007). A new look at habits and the habit-goal interface. *Psychological Review, 114*(4), 843–863. https://doi.org/10.1037/0033-295X.114.4.843

Wood, W., & Neal, D. T. (2016). Healthy through habit: Interventions for initiating & maintaining health behavior change. *Behavioral Science & Policy, 2*(1), 71–83. https://doi.org/10.1353/bsp.2016.0008

Wood, W., & Rünger, D. (2016). Psychology of habit. *Annual Review of Psychology, 67*(1), 289–314. https://doi.org/10.1146/annurev-psych-122414-033417

The Last Chapter (but Not the Last Word) on Deliberate Practice

Sam Malins, Daryl Chow, Scott D. Miller, and Mark A. Hubble

After climbing a great hill, one only finds that there are many more hills to climb.
—NELSON MANDELA

DECISION POINT

Begin here if you have read the book *Better Results* and

- are routinely measuring your performance *and*
- have collected sufficient data to establish a reliable, evidence-based profile of your therapeutic effectiveness *and*
- have completed the Taxonomy of Deliberate Practice Activities in Psychotherapy *and*
- no longer need help leveraging the factors responsible for treatment outcome nor developing a consistent deliberate practice routine.

Above all else, a field guide is supposed to be practical—an accessible, easy-to-use repository of information pertinent to a particular area of interest or subject. It is not a textbook. It is a "ready reference" designed to help the reader quickly find what they want or need to know when they want or need to know it.

In the preceding chapters, leading experts have reviewed and summarized the empirical literature, distilled evidence-based principles, and offered concrete

https://doi.org/10.1037/0000358-010
The Field Guide to Better Results: Evidence-Based Exercises to Improve Therapeutic Effectiveness,
S. D. Miller, D. Chow, S. Malins, and M. A. Hubble (Editors)

exercises you can use to improve your results. The focus is idiographic, not nomothetic—it is focus on you, the individual practitioner, what you can do to improve at a given point in your career; it is your development, not what you are being told to do to be effective (Chow et al., 2022).

The *Field Guide* (*FG*) picks up where *Better Results* left off. Chapter 1, "Identifying Your 'What' to Practice," covered how to determine your specific target for deliberate practice (DP). Chapter 2, "Identifying and Refining Your Individualized Learning Objective," clarified how to break down your target into a series of executable steps, turning hoped-for improvements into well-defined learning goals, along with specific activities designed to promote progress. Chapters 3 through 7 shifted attention to the factors most responsible for change. Which to read will depend on your objective. Need help leveraging client factors? Start with Chapter 3. If your performance data and completed Taxonomy of Deliberate Practice Activities in Psychotherapy (TDPA; Chow & Miller, 2022; see Appendix A, this volume) reveal a deficiency in building hope and an expectation of success, turn to Chapter 6. The same holds for Chapters 4, 5, and 7—you, the therapist, your relationship with your clients, and the structure you bring to your work, respectively. Finally, Chapter 8, "Habits: The Key to a Sustainable System of Deliberate Practice," provided direction for transforming your "good intentions" into a sustainable system of DP.

In content and form, the *FG* leaves room for the novel and unexpected. On your journey, you may not encounter all that is described in the volume. Hopefully, it helps you see and understand what you might otherwise miss and even venture into uncharted territory, making discoveries of your own. Encouraging their readers to explore the unknown when they have a guide for what *is* known has, for example, stretched human understanding of nature and wildlife (Pearson & Shetterly, 2006).

True, the current evidence shows DP is more effective than traditional approaches for teaching and training therapists (Barrett-Naylor et al., 2020; Newman et al., 2022; Westra et al., 2021). Still, much remains unknown and subject to revision; for example,

- how long DP takes to facilitate improvement,
- whether everyone benefits from DP in the same way,
- if certain types of DP plans yield faster and better results (Ericsson & Pool, 2016),
- how to tailor DP to the individual to maximize benefit,
- the characteristics of effective coaches and learning feedback, and
- the environmental conditions (e.g., social support, schedule, intrinsic and extrinsic rewards) most supportive of DP (Clements-Hickman & Reese, 2020).

At the most basic level, agreement about what DP is and what it is not has yet to make its way into the profession. As noted in Chapter 1, some are equating DP with just another way of mastering particular methods and techniques, assuming that doing so will yield better results. It is also noteworthy that no investigation published to date includes a DP condition meeting the four

FIGURE 9.1. The Four Pillars of Deliberate Practice (DP)

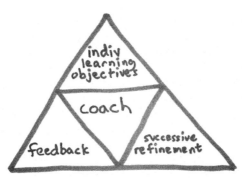

empirically established criteria. As reported in a meta-analysis by Miller et al. (2018), these include (a) an assessment of the performer's baseline ability or skill level against which progress can be determined, (b) corrective feedback targeted to the individual's execution of skills being learned, (c) development of a plan for successive refinement over time, and (d) guidance provided by an expert coach or teacher (see Figure 9.1). Until consensus is reached and qualifying studies are performed, our knowledge remains principally based on naturalistic and retrospective studies. Even then, though desirable, the dominant form of research employed in the field—randomized controlled trials—will likely need to give way to designs congruent with the highly individualized nature of DP. For all these reasons, as with all field guides, this one should be viewed as a "work in progress."

Looking forward, as interest and research on the subject grow, understanding of DP will likely (and hopefully) change and evolve. To ensure DP remains true to Ericsson's discoveries for transforming professional development versus being made a servant of conventional thinking and practices, we believe four points are critical for both clinicians and researchers to keep in mind.

MAKE CLEAR DISTINCTIONS BETWEEN NAIVE, PURPOSEFUL, STRUCTURED, AND DELIBERATE PRACTICE

In their last book, *Peak: Secrets from the New Science in Expertise*, Ericsson and Pool (2016) identified three different types of practice (see Chapter 1): naive, purposeful, and deliberate. A 2019 paper called attention to a fourth: structured (Ericsson & Harwell, 2019). Distinguishing between the various forms was crucial, Ericsson and Pool maintained, because only one was reliably associated with improving *individual* performance.

The "naive" type is what is most commonly associated with the word *practice*. Repetition is seen as the key component, whether playing a sport or learning to drive a car. Unfortunately, Ericsson and Pool (2016) noted, "Research has shown that . . . once a person reaches [an] level of 'acceptable' performance, [more such] 'practice' doesn't lead to improvement" (p. 13). As such, consistent with the literature reviewed in *BR* and this volume, clinical experience would, at best, qualify as an example of "naive practice."

Most psychotherapy workshops and books with "deliberate practice" in their titles would, according to Ericsson and Pool (2016), at best, be examples of either structured or purposeful practice. With regard to the former, the objective is proficiency and competence, achieving a predetermined standard for the execution of a particular skill. It is planned and goal directed and includes feedback and a way to monitor progress but not individualized learning objectives. Studying, attending a workshop, or reading a book would be examples of the latter. Such practice can certainly be planned and goal directed. Without the input of a coach, however, efforts are subject to a number of threats, including self-assessment bias, limitations in the learner's knowledge and ability that impede development, and the absence of expert feedback designed to optimize learning.

Of the four, only DP is individualized, requiring the performer to "constantly try things that are just beyond [their] current abilities" (Ericsson & Pool, 2016, p. 99). For knowledge to advance, the design of future studies must include "bona fide" DP conditions, reflecting the four criteria reported earlier (see Table 9.1).

GET BEYOND "TIME SPENT" FALLACY IN DP

Ever since writer Malcolm Gladwell (2008) coined the term "the 10,000-hour" rule, many have conflated effective DP with the amount of time devoted to the activity. In fact, Ericsson never made such a claim. Yes, the first study of DP in psychotherapy did find the amount of time a therapist devoted to DP was correlated with effectiveness (Chow et al., 2015). However, as everyone learns in their first statistics course, correlation is not causation. In this context, this was confirmed in the meta-analysis by Miller et al. (2018), revealing mere time spent is not a reliable predictor of effective DP. Naturally, DP takes time. By now, it is hopefully clear the quality and characteristics of practice are what matter most (Ericsson, 2008).

TABLE 9.1. Naive, Purposeful, Structured, and Deliberate Practice

	Naive practice	Purposeful practice	Structured practice	Deliberate practice
Guidance from a coach?	N	N	Y	Y
Individualized learning objectives?	N	Y	N	Y
Learning feedback (LF) and performance feedback (PF)?	PF only (if routine outcome measurement is employed)	PF only	PF only	LF & PF
Successive refinement?	N	Y	Y	Y

ADOPT RESEARCH METHODS AND DESIGNS CONGRUENT WITH THE NATURE AND AIMS OF DELIBERATE PRACTICE

Throughout *BR* and the *FG*, the point has repeatedly been made that DP is a long-term process—once more, "a marathon, not a sprint." Unfortunately, most studies published in our field are short in duration. For example, Chow et al.'s (2022) investigations of DP lasted no more than a few hours. What is more, the typical research design employed—the randomized controlled trial—is far more applicable to assessing the type of mastery associated with purposeful practice than the slow, highly individualized growth that is the hallmark of DP. They can be done, but naturalistic, retrospective, mixed methods, and developmental designs have a better chance of capturing the nuance and complexity of DP.

FOCUS ON PRINCIPLES (NOT MODELS AND METHODS)

Models and their associated techniques have a negligible relationship with outcome. For this reason, linking DP—whether in research or training—to particular approaches is senseless. Better to focus on "first principles," defined as the "fundamental proven axioms in the given arena" ("First Principle," 2022, para. 3). The factors at the core of all effective therapy represented in the TDPA and reviewed in detail in Chapters 3 through 7 are exemplary.

The evidence shows that when DP is organized around principles rather than emulating a reference example (i.e., here is how it's done, do it this way), people are better able to transfer what they learn to novel situations (Chow et al., 2022; Haskell, 2001). Thus, instead of testing for the mastery of a particular skill, future research and training programs should assess the degree to which whatever is taught transfers successfully to other clients, contexts, and conditions. After all, as MacKeough and colleagues (1995) noted, "Transfer of learning . . . [is] the ultimate aim of teaching" (p. vii).

CONCLUSION

In the end, the ultimate test of *BR* and the *FG*—the only outcome that matters—is outcome. Administering measures, seeking feedback, regularly scrutinizing our performance, exposing ourselves to critique, pouring over data, and devoting time and resources to completing the exercises in both volumes will all have been for naught unless more of the people who seek your help are being helped. After all, for most of us, that is the reason we chose this profession, our first first principle.

REFERENCES

Barrett-Naylor, R., Malins, S., Levene, J., Biswas, S., Mays, C., & Main, G. (2020). Brief training in psychological assessment and interventions skills for cancer care staff: A mixed methods evaluation of deliberate practice techniques. *Psycho-Oncology, 29*(11), 1786–1793. https://doi.org/10.1002/pon.5393

Chow, D., & Miller, S. D. (2022). *Taxonomy of Deliberate Practice Activities in Psychotherapy—Therapist Version* (Version 6). International Center for Clinical Excellence.

Chow, D. L., Miller, S. D., Seidel, J. A., Kane, R. T., Thornton, J. A., & Andrews, W. P. (2015). The role of deliberate practice in the development of highly effective psychotherapists. *Psychotherapy, 52*(3), 337–345. https://doi.org/10.1037/pst0000015

Chow, L., Miller, K., & Jones, H. (2022). *Improving difficult conversations in therapy: A randomized trial of a deliberate practice training program* [Manuscript submitted for publication]. International Center for Clinical Excellence, Chicago, IL.

Clements-Hickman, A. L., & Reese, R. J. (2020). Improving therapists' effectiveness: Can deliberate practice help? *Professional Psychology: Research and Practice, 51*(6), 606–612. Advance online publication. https://doi.org/10.1037/pro0000318

Ericsson, K. A. (2008). Deliberate practice and acquisition of expert performance: A general overview. *Academic Emergency Medicine, 15*(11), 988–994. https://doi.org/10.1111/j.1553-2712.2008.00227.x

Ericsson, K. A., & Harwell, K. W. (2019). Deliberate practice and proposed limits on the effects of practice on the acquisition of expert performance: Why the original definition matters and recommendations for future research. *Frontiers in Psychology, 10,* 2396. https://doi.org/10.3389/fpsyg.2019.02396

Ericsson, K. A., & Pool, R. (2016). *Peak: Secrets from the science of expertise.* Houghton Mifflin Harcourt.

First principle. (2022, April 25). In *Wikipedia.* https://en.wikipedia.org/wiki/First_principle

Gladwell, M. (2008). *Outliers: The story of success.* Little, Brown and Company.

Haskell, R. E. (2001). *Transfer of learning: Cognition, instruction, and reasoning.* Academic Press. https://doi.org/10.1016/B978-012330595-4/50003-2

MacKeough, A., Lupart, J., & Marini, A. (Eds.). (1995). *Teaching for transfer: Fostering generalization in learning.* Routledge.

Miller, S. D., Chow, D., Wampold, B., Hubble, M. A., Del Re, A. C., Maeschalck, C., & Bargmann, S. (2018). To be or not to be (an expert)? Revisiting the role of deliberate practice in improving performance. *High Ability Studies, 31*(1), 5–15. https://doi.org/10.1080/13598139.2018.1519410

Newman, D. S., Villarreal, J. N., Gerrard, M. K., McIntire, H., Barrett, C. A., & Kaiser, L. T. (2022). Deliberate practice of consultation communication skills: A randomized controlled trial. *School Psychology, 37*(3), 225–235. Advance online publication. https://doi.org/10.1037/spq0000494

Pearson, D. L., & Shetterly, J. A. (2006). How do published field guides influence interactions between amateurs and professionals in entomology? *American Entomologist, 52*(4), 246–252. https://doi.org/10.1093/ae/52.4.246

Westra, H. A., Norouzian, N., Poulin, L., Coyne, A., Constantino, M. J., Hara, K., Olson, D., & Antony, M. M. (2021). Testing a deliberate practice workshop for developing appropriate responsivity to resistance markers. *Psychotherapy, 58*(2), 175–185. https://doi.org/10.1037/pst0000311

Taxonomy of Deliberate Practice Activities in Psychotherapy— Therapist Version (Version 6)

Daryl Chow and Scott D. Miller (© 2015, 2017, 2019, 2022)

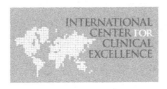

Your Name: _____ **Your Coach's Name:** _____
Date: _____

Objectives:

1. To develop clear and concrete learning objectives specific to the clinical population you work with in order to promote professional development.

2. To establish a baseline of learning goals and to evaluate professional growth routinely (i.e., monthly), in concert with routine outcome monitoring (ROM) practices.

Overview:

There are five broad domains for deliberate practice in psychotherapy:

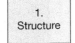 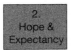 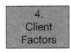 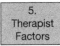

Instructions:

1. **Know Your Work:**

   Begin with regular monitoring of your clinical work using standardized measures of relationship and outcome. Once sufficient data has been collected to establish a reliable, evidence-based profile of your work, identify parameters indicating where your performance falls short of established norms.

   Recall as vividly as possible your clients in the last typical work week (extend to the last 2 work weeks if necessary). To aid with your recall, review audio/video recordings of your sessions.

2. **Rate:**

   Go through the list of activities contained in the TDPA, rating each of them according to your own appraisal of how you perform in each of the domains.

3. **Describe:**

   Put notes in on the last column to add richness and detail to your ratings.

4. **Prioritize:**

   Review the ENTIRE document, identifying the **top 3 activities** you believe will have a significant impact on improving your ability to engage and help your clients. After you have identified your top 3 activities, select **one** to work on.

5. **Compare and Contrast:**

   Enlist a coach, or content-area expert to complete the Coach version of the TDPA. Compare ratings and the top 3 activities. Work together to identify and design a single learning objective.

6. **Consolidate:**

   Complete the final page of the TDPA, **Consolidation,** and

7. **Plan:**

   Develop a routine for reviewing the TDPA periodically (i.e., every month). Expect learning objectives to change and evolve as you make progress.

*Notes: Please select the TOP 3 ACTIVITIES across the entire list (e.g., not necessarily within each of the domains). The three do not have to be the lowest scored item. Complete the consolidation section at the end to help clarify your professional development plan.

TABLE A.1. The Structure Domain of Deliberate Practice Activities

Themes	Activities	Current Rating (0–10)	Select & Rank the TOP 3 Activities to work on*	Notes
	A. How do you start a first session?			
	B. How do you start subsequent sessions?			
1. Structure	C. How do you close a session?			
	D. How do you formally elicit detailed and nuanced feedback at each session?			
	E. How do you integrate the use of feedback measures into your way of working?			

(continues)

TABLE A.1. The Structure Domain of Deliberate Practice Activities (*Continued*)

Themes	Activities	Current Rating (0–10)	Select & Rank the TOP 3 Activities to work on*	Notes
	F. How do you change your way of working in response to client feedback (e.g., the method, the frequency/dose, the provider)?			
	G. How do you prepare for a planned closure of therapy?			
	H. How do you plan and decide on the number and length of sessions you offer?			
	I. How do you share with your client that your work together is unfolding as it should so they know progress is being made toward the resolution of their problem/concern?			
	J. How do you maintain the organization and focus in your work from session to session?			

K. How do you ensure the accuracy and timing of your therapeutic interventions?			
L. How do the methods, techniques, and activities within and outside of formal sessions flow logically from your theory/model for helping clients?			
M. What *structured* procedures do you have for resolving problems in therapy and how do you use them?			
N. How do you balance structure and flexibility in therapeutic boundaries, sequence, and appraisal on the model of therapeutic structure?			
O. How does the space in which you work embody a therapeutic climate (color, furnishings, artwork)?			
P. Others (please describe specifically to structuring the session):			

Note. Please select the TOP 3 ACTIVITIES across the entire list (e.g., not necessarily within each of the domains). The three do not have to be the lowest scored item. Complete the consolidation section at the end to help clarify your professional development plan.

TABLE A.2. The Hope and Expectancy Domain of Deliberate Practice Activities

Themes	Activities	Current Rating (0–10)	Select & Rank the TOP 3 Activities to work on*	Notes
	A. How do you induct clients into therapy? Inform them about what to expect from one session to the next? Explain your respective roles (e.g., client, therapist)?			
	B. How does the explanation you offer for your client's distress engender hope and expectation for change?			
2. Hope & Expectancy	C. How do you persuade the client to have a favorable assessment and acceptance of your clinical rationale and related techniques?			
	D. How do you adapt your treatment rationale to foster client engagement and hope?			
	E. How do you communicate a hopeful and optimistic stance toward your client and their problem/concerns (including capitalizing on times when clients express high hope and expectancy)?			

F. How do you convey a sense of confidence and belief in you and your treatment approach?			
G. How to you measure/assess client hope and expectancy at the outset of and throughout care?			
H. Others (please describe specifically to hope and expectancy):			

Note. Please select the TOP 3 ACTIVITIES across the entire list (e.g., not necessarily within each of the domains). The three do not have to be the lowest scored item. Complete the consolidation section at the end to help clarify your professional development plan.

TABLE A.3. The Relationship Factors Domain of Deliberate Practice Activities

Themes	Activities	Current Rating (0–10)	Select & Rank the TOP 3 Activities to work on*	Notes
	i. How do you establish goal consensus in the first/subsequent sessions?			
	ii. How do you help a client who has no clear goals in therapy?			
3. Relationship A. Effective Focus	iii. How do you mobilize clients' willingness to engage in a therapeutic process/ activity?			
	iv. How do you encourage your client to confront, experience, or deal with difficult topics or problems?			

i. How do you explicitly convey warmth, understanding, acceptance, and positive regard toward your client?				
ii. How do you promote emotional engagement/safety?				
iii. How do you foster a sense of mutuality with your client (e.g., responsiveness, feelings, expectations, reciprocity)?				
iv. How do you remain true to yourself and in the interaction with your client?				
v. How do you explicitly communicate empathic attunement?				
vi. How do you deepen your client's emotional experiencing?				

3. Relationship

B. The Impact Factor

(continues)

TABLE A.3. The Relationship Factors Domain of Deliberate Practice Activities (*Continued*)

Themes	Activities	Current Rating (0–10)	Select & Rank the TOP 3 Activities to work on*	Notes
3. Relationship C. Motivation	i. How do you assess and work with a client's readiness for change?			
	ii. How do you increase homework compliance?			
3. Relationship D. Difficulties	i. How do you deal with ruptures in the alliance?			
	ii. How do you deal with an angry client?			
	iii. How do you deal with a client who is feeling hopeless?			

iv. How do you deal with strong and difficult emotions arising in the session?		
v. How do you manage a client who is at high risk of suicide?		
vi. How do you manage a client mandated for treatment?		
vii. Others (please describe specifically to alliance factors):		

*Note. Please select the TOP 3 ACTIVITIES across the entire list (e.g., not necessarily within each of the domains). The three do not have to be the lowest scored item. Complete the consolidation section at the end to help clarify your professional development plan.

TABLE A.4. The Client Factors Domain of Deliberate Practice Activities

Themes	Activities	Current Rating (0–10)	Select & Rank the TOP 3 Activities to work on*	Notes
	A. Prior to initiating treatment, how do you actively and directly prepare your client for what will happen while they are in care?			
	B. How do you learn about your client's expectations regarding treatment and their role in the process?			
4. Client Factors	C. How to you actively tailor the type, intensity, and nature of treatment interventions to fit the client's level of interest, engagement, and relational style throughout (and at each session of) treatment?			
	D. How do you incorporate your client's strengths, abilities, and resources into care?			

E. How do you incorporate your client's values, beliefs (including but not limited to religious and spiritual), and cultural systems into care?		
F. How do you actively utilize extratherapeutic events (positive and negative) to influence participation and progress?		
G. How do you incorporate or help the client build their social support network?		
H. Others (please describe specifically to client factors):		

Note. Please select the TOP 3 ACTIVITIES across the entire list (e.g., not necessarily within each of the domains). The three do not have to be the lowest scored item. Complete the consolidation section at the end to help clarify your professional development plan.

TABLE A.5. The Therapist Factors Domain of Deliberate Practice Activities

Themes	Activities	Current Rating (0–10)	Select & Rank the TOP 3 Activities to work on*	Notes
	i. How do you regulate your anxiety when encountering a difficult interaction with a client?			
	ii. How do you manage negative feelings toward your client (e.g., anger, discouragement, hostility, blame)?			
5. Therapist A. The Use of the Self	iii. How do you maintain appropriate boundaries and roles with your clients (e.g., not letting personal emotions or life events bleed into/ affect your clinical work)?			
	iv. How do you remain reflective versus reactive in session with clients?			
	v. How do you utilize self-disclosure?			

vi. How do you integrate your life experiences, identity, and self into your personal clinical style?			
vii. How do you operationalize empirically supported principles of effective clinical work in a way unique to you as a person?			
viii. How do you find the right words at the right time or in the right situation?			
5. Therapist i. How do you engage in solitary deliberate practice *outside of* sessions in your typical work week?			
B. Outside of Sessions ii. Others (please describe specifically to therapist factors):			

Note. Please select the TOP 3 ACTIVITIES across the entire list (e.g., not necessarily within each of the domains). The three do not have to be the lowest scored item. Complete the consolidation section at the end to help clarify your professional development plan.

CONSOLIDATION:

Instructions:

1. The **Top 3 Activities** to work on from the taxonomy are your **Stretch Goals.** They are the objectives at the margin of your "zone of proximal development." List them in order of priority. Once listed, choose **ONE** to focus on in deliberate practice. Recall, to improve results, your one identified stretch goal must be associated with treatment outcome. Consult the research evidence to confirm (see https://darylchow.com/frontiers/what-are-the-perennial-pillars-for-psychotherapists/ for some examples).

2. Discrepancies are likely to exist between the goals you and your coach identify and are a good place to begin dialogue. Choosing and refining learning objectives is an iterative process. Revise until agreement is reached that fits your interests and your coach or supervisor's knowledge and skills.

3. State your chosen stretch goal in **"SMART"** terms (**S**pecific, **M**easurable, **A**chievable, **R**elevant, **T**ime bound) to assist you in identifying concrete activities you can engage in to reach your stretch goal.

4. Review your Stretch and SMART Goals on an ongoing basis, also setting aside a specific date and time to review your progress. Check for impact on your performance metrics.

Current Date: _____   Review Date: _____

TABLE A.6. Consolidation of Stretch and Smart Goals

S/N	STRETCH GOAL (Your current identified "Top 3 Activities" to work on)	SMART GOAL (Specific, Measurable, Achievable, Relevant, Time bound)	Review & Reflect
1			
2			
3			

Taxonomy of Deliberate Practice Activities in Psychotherapy Exercise Guide

Exercises in *The Field Guide* are linked to the five factors having leverage on the outcome psychotherapy. Once you have collected sufficient data to establish a reliable, evidence-based profile of your therapeutic effectiveness, completed the Taxonomy of Deliberate Practice Activities in Psychotherapy, and narrowed your focus to a single learning objective, this guide may be used to quickly locate applicable exercises.

TABLE B.1. Structure Activities

Themes	Activities	Chapter	Exercise number	Page/s
	A. How do you start a first session?	6 7	5 1, 2, 5	147 167, 168, 172
	B. How do you start subsequent sessions?	7	1, 2	167, 168
1. Structure	C. How do you close a session?	7	1, 2	167, 168
	D. How do you formally elicit detailed and nuanced feedback at each session?	5 6 7	8 2 1, 6	125 145 167, 174
	E. How do you integrate the use of feedback measures into your way of working?	4 5 6 7	4 7 1, 2 1, 6	97 124 144, 145 167, 174

F. How do you change your way of working in response to client feedback (e.g., the method, the frequency/dose, the provider)?	4 5 6 7	4 7, 8 1, 2, 4, 5 1, 4, 5, 6	97 124, 125 144, 145, 147, 147 167, 171, 172, 174
G. How do you prepare for a planned closure of therapy?	6 7	3 1, 5	146 167, 172
H. How do you plan and decide on the number and length of sessions you offer?	5 6 7	8 1 1, 4, 5	125 144 167, 171, 172
I. How do you share with your client that your work together is unfolding as it should so they know progress is being made toward the resolution of their problem/concern?	5 7	8 1, 3, 4	125 167, 171, 171
J. How do you maintain the organization and focus in your work from session to session?	4 7	4 1, 3, 4, 5	97 167, 171, 171, 172
K. How do you ensure the accuracy and timing of your therapeutic interventions?	5 6 7	6 5 1, 3, 4	123 147 167, 171, 171

(continues)

TABLE B.1. Structure Activities (*Continued*)

Themes	Activities	Chapter	Exercise number	Page/s
	L. How do the methods, techniques, and activities within and outside of formal sessions flow logically from your theory/model for helping clients?	7	1	167
	M. What *structured* procedures do you have for resolving problems in therapy and how do you use them?	7	1	167
	N. How do you balance structure and flexibility in therapeutic boundaries, sequence, and appraisal on the model of therapeutic structure?	7	1	167
	O. How does the space in which you work embody a therapeutic climate (color, furnishings, artwork)?			
	P. Others (please describe specifically to structuring the session):			

TABLE B.2. Hope and Expectancy Activities

Themes	Activities	Chapter	Exercise number	Page/s
	A. How do you induct clients into therapy? Inform them about what to expect from one session to the next? Explain your respective roles (e.g., client, therapist)?	6	1, 2, 5	144, 145, 147
	B. How does the explanation you offer for your client's distress engender hope and expectation for change?	5 6	8 1, 4, 5, 6	125 144, 147, 147, 149
2. Hope & Expectancy	C. How do you persuade the client to have a favorable assessment and acceptance of your clinical rationale and related techniques?	6	4, 5, 6	147, 147, 149
	D. How do you adapt your treatment rationale to foster client engagement and hope?	4 6	4 3, 4, 6	97 146, 147, 149
	E. How do you communicate a hopeful and optimistic stance toward your client and their problem/concerns (including capitalizing on times when clients express high hope and expectancy)?	6	3, 5, 6, 7	146, 147, 149, 149

(continues)

TABLE B.2. Hope and Expectancy Activities (*Continued*)

Themes	Activities	Chapter	Exercise number	Page/s
	F. How do you convey a sense of confidence and belief in you and your treatment approach?	6	3, 5, 6, 7	146, 147, 149, 149
	G. How to you measure/assess client hope and expectancy at the outset of and throughout care?	6	1, 2, 5, 6, 7	144, 145, 146, 149, 149
	H. Others (please describe specifically to hope and expectancy):			

TABLE B.3. Relationship Factors Activities

Themes	Activities	Chapter	Exercise number	Page/s
	i. How do you establish goal consensus in the first/subsequent sessions?	5	7, 8	124, 125
	ii. How do you help a client who has no clear goals in therapy?	5	7, 8	124, 125
3. Relationship A. Effective Focus	iii. How do you mobilize clients' willingness to engage in a therapeutic process/activity?	5 6	1, 7 1, 2, 3, 4	118, 124 144, 145, 146, 147
	iv. How do you encourage your client to confront, experience, or deal with difficult topics or problems?	2 5 6	1 1, 7 1, 2, 6	34 118, 124 144, 145

(continues)

TABLE B.3. Relationship Factors Activities (Continued)

Themes	Activities	Chapter	Exercise number	Page/s
	i. How do you explicitly convey warmth, understanding, acceptance, and positive regard toward your client?	3 4 5 6	1, 2 1, 2, 3, 5 1, 2, 4 1	66, 67 94, 95, 96, 98 118, 119, 121 144
	ii. How do you promote emotional engagement/safety?	3 4 5	1, 2 1, 2, 3, 5 1, 4, 6, 9	66, 67 94, 95, 96, 98 118, 121, 123, 126
	iii. How do you foster a sense of mutuality with your client (e.g., responsiveness, feelings, expectations, reciprocity)?	4 5	3 1, 3, 5, 6	96 118, 120, 122, 123
3. Relationship B. The Impact Factor	iv. How do you remain true to yourself and in the interaction with your client?	2 4 5 6	1 2 1, 5, 6 6, 7	34 95 118, 122, 123 149, 149
	v. How do you explicitly communicate empathic attunement?	3 4 5	1 2, 3 2, 3	66 95, 96 119, 120
	vi. How do you deepen your client's emotional experiencing?	4	2, 3	95, 96

3. Relationship C. Motivation	i. How do you assess and work with a client's readiness for change?	3 6	2 6	67 149
	ii. How do you increase homework compliance?	5	7	124
	i. How do you deal with ruptures in the alliance?	4 5	1, 2, 3, 5 1, 9	94, 95, 96, 98 118, 126
	ii. How do you deal with an angry client?	4	1, 2, 3, 5	94, 95, 96, 98
3. Relationship D. Difficulties	iii. How do you deal with a client who is feeling hopeless?	4 6	1, 5 2, 5	94, 98 145, 147
	iv. How do you deal with strong and difficult emotions arising in the session?	4 5 6	1, 2, 5 1 3	94, 95, 98 118 146

(continues)

TABLE B.3. Relationship Factors Activities (*Continued*)

Themes	Activities	Chapter	Exercise number	Page/s
	v. How do you manage a client who is at high risk of suicide?			
	vi. How do you manage a client mandated for treatment?			
	vii. Others (please describe specifically to alliance factors):			

TABLE B.4. Client Factors Activities

Themes	Activities	Chapter	Exercise number	Page/s
	A. Prior to initiating treatment, how do you actively and directly prepare your client for what will happen while they are in care?	3	2	67
		5	7, 8	124, 125
		6	1, 2, 5, 6, 7	144, 145, 147, 149, 149
	B. How do you learn about your client's expectations regarding treatment and their role in the process?	3	2, 6	67, 71
		4	1	94
		5	7, 8	124, 125
		6	2, 6	145, 149
4. Client Factors	C. How to you actively tailor the type, intensity, and nature of treatment interventions to fit the client's level of interest, engagement, and relational style throughout (and at each session of) treatment?	3	1, 3, 5, 6	66, 68, 70, 71
		4	1, 4, 5	94, 97, 98
		5	2, 3	119, 120
		6	6	149
	D. How do you incorporate your client's strengths, abilities, and resources into care?	4	1	94
		5	3, 4	120, 121
	E. How do you incorporate your client's values, beliefs (including but not limited to religious and spiritual), and cultural systems into care?	3	1, 2, 3, 4, 5	66, 67, 68, 69, 70
		4	2	95
		5	3, 7, 8	120, 124, 125
		6	1	144

(continues)

TABLE B.4. Client Factors Activities (*Continued*)

Themes	Activities	Chapter	Exercise number	Page/s
	F. How do you actively utilize extratherapeutic events (positive and negative) to influence participation and progress?	3	1, 6, 7	66, 68, 71
	G. How do you incorporate or help the client build their social support network?			
	H. Others (please describe specifically to client factors):			

TABLE B.5. Therapist Factors Activities

Themes	Activities	Chapter	Exercise number	Page/s
	i. How do you regulate *your* anxiety when encountering a difficult interaction with a client?	3 4 5	1 1, 2, 4, 5 6, 9	66 94, 95, 97, 98 123, 126
	ii. How do you manage negative feelings toward your client (e.g., anger, discouragement, hostility, blame)?	3 4 5 6	1, 4, 7 1, 2, 5 4, 6, 9 4, 7	66, 69, 71 94, 95, 98 121, 123, 126 147, 149
5. Therapist A. The Use of the Self	iii. How do you maintain appropriate boundaries and roles with your clients (e.g., not letting personal emotions or life events bleed into/affect your clinical work)?	3 4	7 1, 2	71 94, 95
	iv. How do you remain reflective versus reactive in session with clients?	3 4 5 6	1, 4, 5, 7 1, 2, 3, 5 3, 9 4, 7	66, 69, 70, 71 94, 95, 96, 98 120, 126 147, 149
	v. How do you utilize self-disclosure?	4	2	95

(continues)

TABLE B.5. Therapist Factors Activities (Continued)

Themes	Activities	Chapter	Exercise number	Page/s
	vi. How do you integrate your life experiences, identity, and self into your personal clinical style?	2	1	35
	vii. How do you operationalize empirically supported principles of effective clinical work in a way unique to you as a person?	3 4	3 3	68 96
	viii. How do you find the right words at the right time or in the right situation?	3 4 5	5, 6 2, 3 3	70, 71 95, 96 120
	i. How do you engage in solitary deliberate practice outside of sessions in your typical work week?	3 5	1, 3, 4, 5 3	66, 68, 69, 70 120
5. Therapist B. Outside of Sessions	ii. Others (please describe specifically to therapist factors):			

INDEX

A

Abilities of client, incorporating, 218, 235
Abraham, C., 198
Abstraction, levels of, 19–21, 56
Acceptance
  conveying, 215, 232
  of treatment rationale, 212, 229
Accomplishments, reflecting on, 21
Accuracy, of interventions, 211, 227
Action stage, 54, 55
Active rest, 190–191
Activities of therapy, flow to, 211, 228
Addressing Correlates of Client OE
    (Exercise 6), 149
Aderka, I. M., 62
Adherence
  to treatment manuals, 84, 111, 163
  to treatment model, 91, 160
Adolescents
  alliance with, 115–117
  therapeutic structure for, 158
Adult psychotherapy, alliance in, 115
Affect, focusing on, 160
Affirmation, 112–114
"African American," use of term, 51
Age
  client's, 49, 134, 136–142
  correlation of OE with, 136
  and strength of OE–outcome association,
    134, 141–142
  therapist's, 88, 89
Alcoholics Anonymous, 61

Alignment
  with client, 117, 119–122, 124–126
  of identity and objectives, 185–186
Al-Krenawi, A., 176
All Change (Exercise 5), 187, 190
Alliance, 115–116. *See also* Therapeutic
    alliance
  adjusting work to improve, 96–97
  in adult psychotherapy, 115
  defined, 115
  humility and, 85
  and OE–outcome association, 134–136,
    142
  real relationship vs., 114
  as relationship factor, 112
  ruptures in. *See* Ruptures in alliance
  sustainable use of metrics for, 174–175
  in youth psychotherapy, 115–116
Allowing for Differences (Exercise 5), 70
Alternative Descriptions (Exercise 1),
    66–67
American Psychological Association (APA),
    15
American Psychologist, 9
Ametrano, R. M., 137, 150
Anderson, Timothy, 85
Angry clients, 216, 233
Anticipation, 186
Antigoals (Exercise 5), 37, 42
Anxiety, regulation of, 220, 237
Anxious attachment style, 56, 57

ABOUT THE EDITORS

Scott D. Miller, PhD, is the founder of the International Center for Clinical Excellence, an international consortium of clinicians, researchers, and educators dedicated to promoting excellence in behavioral health services. Dr. Miller conducts workshops and training in the United States and abroad, helping hundreds of agencies and organizations, public and private, to achieve superior results. He is one of a handful of "invited faculty" whose work, thinking, and research are featured at the prestigious "Evolution of Psychotherapy" conference. He is the author, editor, and coauthor of scores of professional and research articles and 15 books, including *The Heart and Soul of Change: What Works in Therapy* and *Better Results: Using Deliberate Practice to Improve Therapeutic Effectiveness.*

Daryl Chow, PhD, is a practicing psychologist and trainer. He published the first empirical study of deliberate practice in psychotherapy. His books include *The Write to Recovery: Personal Stories and Lessons About Recovery From Mental Health Concerns, The First Kiss: Undoing the Intake Model and Igniting First Sessions in Psychotherapy,* and *Better Results: Using Deliberate Practice to Improve Therapeutic Effectiveness.* His website, Frontiers of Psychotherapist Development (https://darylchow.com/frontiers/), is aimed at inspiring and sustaining practitioners' professional and personal development.

Sam Malins, PhD, is a clinical psychologist working on the integration of physical and mental health care at Nottinghamshire Healthcare NHS Foundation Trust and the University of Nottingham. He works clinically in cancer care. His research focuses on ways to enhance psychological care across settings, often using digital technology. He is currently a National Institute for Health and Care Research clinical lecturer in the Integrated Clinical Academic Programme and is working on methods to help psychological therapists improve their effectiveness.

Mark A. Hubble, PhD, graduated from the prestigious postdoctoral fellowship in clinical psychology at Menninger and is a founding member of the International Center for Clinical Excellence. He formerly served as a contributing editor for the then *Family Therapy Networker* and as editor for the *Journal of Systemic Therapies*. With Scott Miller, he has coauthored or coedited eight books, numerous book chapters, peer-reviewed articles and research, and various commentaries. Their bestselling volume (with Barry Duncan), *The Heart and Soul of Change: What Works in Therapy,* earned the Menninger Alumni Association Scientific Writing Award. Dr. Hubble's scholarship extends to the transtheoretical curative factors in psychotherapy, data-based outcome management systems, and excellence in clinical practice.